OTHER VOLUMES IN
EXERCISES IN DIAGNOSTIC RADIOLOGY

Published

Volume 1—Squire, Colaiace and Strutynsky: *The Chest*
Volume 2—Squire, Colaiace and Strutynsky: *The Abdomen*
Volume 3—Squire, Colaiace and Strutynsky: *Bone*
Volume 4—Squire, Dreyfuss, Langston, Novelline: *The Total Patient*

Forthcoming

James and Squire: *Nuclear Radiology*
Squire, Strutynsky and Colaiace: *Special Procedures*

EXERCISES IN DIAGNOSTIC RADIOLOGY

5

PEDIATRICS

RICHARD M. HELLER, M.D.

Assistant Professor of Radiology
and Pediatrics,
The Johns Hopkins School of Medicine
Radiologist,
The Johns Hopkins Hospital,
Baltimore, Maryland

LUCY FRANK SQUIRE, M.D.

Professor of Radiology, Downstate
Medical Center, Brooklyn, New York
Consultant in Radiology, Massachusetts General Hospital,
Boston, Massachusetts

W. B. SAUNDERS COMPANY • PHILADELPHIA • LONDON • TORONTO

W. B. Saunders Company: West Washington Square
Philadelphia, Pa. 19105

12 Dyott Street
London, WC1A 1DB

833 Oxford Street
Toronto 18, Ontario

Exercises in Diagnostic Radiology – Volume 5 Pediatrics   ISBN 0-7216-4630-1

Print No.:   9   8   7   6   5   4   3   2

PREFACE

Children are not just small adults. They do have some of the diseases of adults, to be sure, although even these tend to be altered by the growth and metabolism peculiar to childhood. In addition there is a spectrum of disease conditions limited to the pediatric age group with its own radiologic patterns, evolving in our understanding as the subspecialty, pediatric radiology. It is as complex and as fascinating as the general field of radiology or any of its other subspecialties.

Several decades ago, the superb textbook of Dr. John Caffey appeared (*Pediatric X-Ray Diagnosis*, published by Year Book), and has ever since led the field as an encyclopedic teaching and reference work. The authors' intention in producing this little volume is to present in problem format some of the highlights of the pediatric radiologic discipline. The problems and answers are offered to medical students, pediatric house officers, and radiology residents with the conviction that the subjects chosen are suitable for inclusion in board examinations and are common enough to be recognized at the end of training in either pediatrics or general radiology.

A conscious attempt has been made not to duplicate material already presented in the earlier volumes of this series, particularly in the section on Bone Growth in Volume 3. As indicated in the table of contents, the book is subdivided into groups of problems relating to the pediatric chest, abdomen, brain, and bones. Names and some details of the presenting histories have been altered, but the clinical facts of the cases are true.

As with the other volumes, we will be grateful for ideas and suggestions from our readers.

RICHARD M. HELLER

Department of Radiology
The Johns Hopkins Hospital
Baltimore, Maryland

ACKNOWLEDGMENTS

The authors most gratefully acknowledge their debt to the late Dr. John Hope, not only for helpful advice and exquisite case material originally given to one of us (LFS), but also for the example of his way of doing things, long an inspiration to us and to so many others in his field.

We are also profoundly indebted to Dr. Edward B. D. Neuhauser and the group of radiologists surrounding him at the Children's Hospital Medical Center in Boston. Dr. N. Thorne Griscom of that group has reviewed the manuscript, while on vacation. We know of no way to express adequately our gratitude for so generous a gesture or for the comfort of knowing he has checked our material, making a meticulous survey, page by page, and numerous excellent suggestions for improvement. The quality of his kind of editing has been an immeasurable help to us.

Dr. Martin Donner, Chairman of the Department of Radiology at The Johns Hopkins Hospital committed department funds for the preparation of the manuscript and has been a great source of inspiration. Dr. John Dorst's encouragement and advice have been invaluable, and we have drawn on his excellent teaching file for some of the case material used here.

The diagrams and drawings were prepared by Mr. Joseph Dieter, Jr. Our friends at the Eastman Kodak Company, particularly Mrs. Alice Russell and Mr. Thomas Callear, helped by supplying us with a number of glossy prints and permission to reprint some of Dr. Hope's material. Dr. Robert E. Gross and the W. B. Saunders Company have allowed us to reprint Figures 34 and 35 from The Surgery of Infancy and Childhood.

The manuscript was typed by Mrs. Margie Walker.

Many of the photographs were prepared by Henri Hessels and Willie Ragsdale, to whom we are extremely grateful.

Finally, we appreciate the continuous consideration and address to problems which have always been shown us by Mr. John Hanley and Mr. Al Beringer of the W. B. Saunders Company. Authors are fortunate to have such men as publishers.

RMH

LFS

CONTENTS

PREFACE v

ACKNOWLEDGMENTS... vii

CHEST... 1

ABDOMEN 37

SKULL... 93

BONE 119

QUIZ 149

CHEST

TWO PATIENTS WITH DIETARY INDISCRETION

FIGURE 1. Rusty N.

FIGURE 2. Rusty N.

Rusty N., a 3 year old girl, is brought by her mother to the Emergency Room because of a cough of three weeks' duration. This cough is worse at night, keeping the mother awake. Her mother wants *Rusty* to have a shot of penicillin and some cough medicine.

Physical examination shows reduced breath sounds in the distribution of the right lower lobe and right middle lobe. No rales are heard, but there are rhonchi present. Her temperature is normal. You send *Rusty* to the radiology department for PA and lateral chest radiographs.

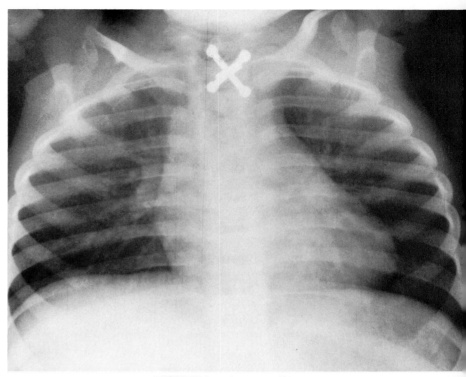

FIGURE 3. Jacques Pierre

Jacques Pierre Perdu, the son of a French Minister without portfolio, is referred to you with the chief complaint of having swallowed a toy. The boy speaks no English. The father speaks and understands English perfectly but, being French, refuses to acknowledge this ability. Your college French helps a little, and you learn that the boy threw a jackstone into the air and caught it in his mouth. This was one hour ago, and since then the jackstone hasn't been seen.

Physical examination is negative, and you decide to request radiographs of the chest, thinking that if the toy isn't seen, you may have to obtain views of the neck and abdomen.

FIGURE 4. Jacques Pierre

ANSWERS

Rusty's chest radiographs show a nail directed vertically and toward the right. Its position so far off the midline indicates that it's not in the esophagus, but instead is in the trachea and right main stem bronchus. The lateral view is not straight, and you can see that one bronchus is normal and the other needs rust inhibitor. The lateral view also shows increased radiodensity in the right middle lobe area, and you can only see one hemidiaphragm. This indicates that the nail must be occluding the intermediate bronchus to the right middle and right lower lobes, resulting in atelectasis of these lobes. The right upper lobe bronchus must be patent, otherwise there would be complete atelectasis of the right lung.

Bronchoscopy was performed and the nail removed. Unfortunately, over the next several months *Rusty* had recurrent pneumonias in the areas that had been atelectatic. The child stopped gaining weight and growing. During one of her asymptomatic periods, it was elected to perform a bronchogram (Fig. 5).

This study shows cylindrical dilation of the right lower and middle lobe bronchi. In the right upper lobe bronchus there is the normal tapering of the bronchi as they progress toward the periphery of the lung.

The dilation of the bronchi, or bronchiectasis, is the result of obstruction of the bronchi, stasis of secretions, and infection which destroys the bronchial walls.

If the changes in the bronchi are mild, and the obstruction is relieved promptly, the bronchiectasis may be reversible. *Rusty's* bronchiectasis was too advanced, and a right middle and right lower lobectomy had to be performed. She has done well since surgery and has exhibited normal growth and development.

FIGURE 5. Rusty N.

Jacques Pierre Perdu has "swallowed" a jackstone. On the AP radiograph the tracheal air shadow is to the right of the jackstone. The lateral view shows the jackstone extending posterior to the tracheal air column. These findings indicate that the foreign body is in the esophagus rather than the trachea. It was easily removed using esophagoscopy.

TWO CHILDREN WITH RESPIRATORY DISTRESS

Edward G. is a 3 year old with hoarseness and increasing dyspnea for 24 hours. Currently the child has a temperature of 103°, retraction of the ribs during inspiration, and an inspiratory crow. The boy is not cyanotic, but he seems to have great difficulty breathing, mainly during the inspiratory phase.

FIGURE 6.   Edward G.

Thomas P., also 3 years old, had become suddenly ill earlier the same day with a sore throat, temperature of 105°, and severe inspiratory dyspnea. Physical examination shows redness of the posterior oropharynx and surrounding tissues.

You decide that a chest film is indicated and send *Thomas P.* to the radiology department.

FIGURE 7.   Thomas P.

ANSWERS

Edward G. has croup, or laryngotracheobronchitis. Notice the narrowing of the upper trachea caused by edema and inflammation of the area of the trachea just below the vocal cords, the conus elasticus.

Croup is usually caused by a virus and is frequently preceded by a history of an upper respiratory infection. It occurs in children from age 6 months to 3 years and is usually adequately treated with moist, cool air. Oxygen is added occasionally, but rarely is the disease severe enough to warrant tracheostomy.

This particular child had an additional problem which is illustrated in Figure 8.

Edward G. became increasingly ill as he was observed in the Emergency Ward. It was difficult to examine him, but the tip of the epiglottis was seen to have a "cherry-red color." Clinically, the condition of the child was deteriorating rapidly with the onset of dysphagia, slight cyanosis, restlessness, and a more "toxic" appearance.

A lateral view of the airway was obtained to evaluate the area that couldn't be seen during physical examination.

What's the diagnosis?

Thomas P. has tonsillitis. The radiograph of his trachea is normal and shows the "square shoulders" of the normal subglottic space. If *Thomas* had been in a good mood, he might have cooperated enough to phonate on command, which would have shown apposition of the true vocal cords, the structures which cast the shadows of the "square shoulders." This technique can be used to demonstrate paralyzed vocal cords.

Thomas had a throat culture which produced normal flora. He was not treated with antibiotics and returned to his normal activity of "beating-up" his little sister.

FIGURE 8. Edward G.

Karen A. is a 9 month old patient who was admitted to the hospital because of suspected aspiration of a tin sailboat.

FIGURE 9.   Karen A.

Myrna B. is a 10 month old girl who was quite ill with a temperature of 105.8° and difficulty in breathing associated with noisy respiration.

FIGURE 10.   Myrna B.

Edward's film shows the swollen, "thumb-like" appearance of the epiglottis. This is the structure seen above and behind the hyoid bones. It normally has a smooth and slender appearance as that seen in Figure 9.

Edward has acute epiglottitis in addition to his croup. This combination is rather unusual.

Acute epiglottitis is commonly a more fulminating condition than croup. The onset of the symptoms is sudden and may progress to respiratory obstruction requiring tracheostomy in a matter of hours. Usually, the child complains of intense sore throat and refuses to swallow.

A patient with these symptoms and a fulminating clinical course should have only a limited physical examination of the posterior oropharynx. If the patient is forced to have a thorough examination, this alone may cause obstruction of the airway. Likewise, he should not be forced to lie down for the lateral radiograph of the neck; this, too, may precipitate airway obstruction, and there is no reason why the child should not be sitting in the upright position for the lateral view of the neck.

Treatment will depend upon the degree of respiratory embarrassment. Usually the child is hospitalized so that tracheostomy may be readily performed if necessary. A culture of the epiglottis will commonly demonstrate *Haemophilus influenzae*, although less commonly beta-hemolytic streptococcus and pneumococcus are isolated.

In *Edward's* case, simply cool, moist air and antibiotic therapy were sufficient. He did not require a tracheostomy and after several days in the hospital was discharged feeling fairly well. His culture produced *Haemophilus influenzae*.

Karen A., who was thought to have aspirated a tin sailboat (Fig. 9), was found to have bread crumbs in the trachea. This radiograph was obtained after removal of the bread crumbs and is normal. Notice the slender epiglottis and the horizontal sliver of air beneath the hyoid bone. This is the air in the laryngeal ventricle between the true and false vocal cords.

Compare the width of the tissues anterior to the vertebral bodies in Figure 9 with the same area in Figure 10. *Myrna* has a retropharyngeal abscess. Initially this child had an upper respiratory infection with suppuration of the retropharyngeal lymph nodes. Commonly, dysphagia and dyspnea occur, associated with enlarged cervical lymph nodes and anterior bulging of the posterior pharyngeal wall. Careful fluoroscopy can be used to document thickness of the prevertebral soft tissues. This may be important because expiration, flexion of the neck, and crying will exaggerate *normal* soft tissue thickness. Fluoroscopy of several swallows of barium will help to differentiate the normal retropharyngeal soft tissues from displacement of the esophagus due to a retropharyngeal abscess. The treatment includes antibiotic therapy and surgical drainage.

NORMAL EPIGLOTTIS

POST   ANT

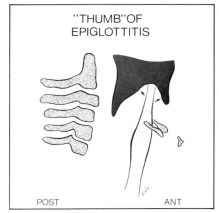

"THUMB" OF EPIGLOTTITIS

POST   ANT

The normal and swollen epiglottis

FIGURE 11. Tammy G.

PROBLEM

Tammy G., a 3 year old girl, is brought to the hospital with a history of repeated colds.

FIGURE 12. Tammy G.

ANSWER

Tammy G. has virtually no symptoms. Her mother noticed that it took longer for her to "throw off a cold" than for her brothers and sister. Imagine everyone's surprise when the chest radiograph revealed the huge mass that we see in Figures 11 and 12. There are several clues involved in the correct interpretation of these radiographs, and they must all be utilized in order to arrive at a reasonable differential diagnosis of this lesion.

In the first place, it would be helpful to decide whether this mass is more likely to be located in the lung or in the mediastinum. Notice that on the lateral view, the anterior lung-mass interface makes an acute angle with the sternum. This usually suggests that the mass is extrapleural, compressing normal lung tissue and causing the plate-like atelectasis seen just beneath the mass against the minor fissure. If this is a mediastinal mass, localization into the proper compartment of the mediastinum should lead to a differential diagnosis that includes certain possibilities and makes other conditions less likely.

Now note that in Figure 13 the barium-opacified esophagus is deviated to the left (the patient's left). Since the esophagus is a posterior mediastinal structure, this mass at least extends into the posterior mediastinum and may originate there. The most common masses arising in the posterior mediastinum are neurogenic tumors. [In the middle mediastinum, foregut duplications including those related to the gut and lung occur in children. In the anterior mediastinum, several diseases present as mass lesions including teratomas, lymphomas, and cystic hygromas as well as thymomas.]

Now observe in Figure 14 the erosion of the posterior portion of the second rib and widening of the second intercostal space. This tells you that this mass has developed slowly, because it takes time for such a rib deformity to develop. So, this is a mass lesion, probably arising in the mediastinum rather than the lung, and probably arising in the posterior mediastinum. It has been present for a long time and suggests a tumor of neurogenic origin.

This little girl had a thoracotomy and resection of the mass. It was, indeed, an extrapleural posterior mediastinal mass which proved to be a ganglioneuroma. These are tumors which arise from the spinal nerves and can invade the spinal canal; thus, any evidence of destruction of the vertebrae or pedicles (or symptoms or physical findings of spinal cord involvement) is an indication for a myelogram. In this case there was no spinal cord involvement, and since surgery this child has had an uncomplicated recovery.

FIGURE 13.   Tammy G.

FIGURE 14.   Tammy G.

THREE CHILDREN SENT TO RADIOLOGY FOR EVALUATION OF "URI'S"

FIGURE 15.
Shadrach

FIGURE 16.
Meshach

FIGURE 17. Abednego

Here are three patients named **Shadrach** (Fig. 15), **Meshach** (Fig. 16), and **Abednego** (Figs. 17 and 18). They all have "URI'S," or upper respiratory infections. Chest radiographs are being made to rule out pneumonia.

FIGURE 18. Abednego

ANSWERS

Shadrach and *Meshach* are the same patient, an 18 month old boy examined because of suspected upper respiratory infection. Why does the mediastinum appear wider in *Shadrach*, and what about the mass extending into the right lung field?

This is the appearance of the normal thymus gland on an expiratory radiograph. Note that you can only count eight ribs posteriorly. Now look at *Meshach*'s radiograph. It was made 30 seconds later but was taken during inspiration and shows nine ribs posteriorly. On this radiograph the thymus appears much smaller and is seen overlying the right main pulmonary artery.

Figure 15 was obtained during expiration and demonstrates the "thymic sail sign." This is the projection of the *normal* thymus into the minor fissure of the right lung. Sometimes indentation upon the thymus by the anterior ribs or costal cartilage creates a rippled appearance that has been termed the "thymic wave sign."

Abednego's chest films (Figs. 17 and 18) show a prominent left hilum with a streaky infiltrate radiating into the left upper lobe. On the lateral film there is a fullness of the hilar region suggesting that the infiltrate in the left upper lobe is accompanied by enlargement of hilar lymph nodes.

This complex of findings should suggest the possibility of primary tuberculosis. The child usually has only nonspecific symptoms such as cough, fever, and sometimes weight loss and lethargy. The radiographic features of primary tuberculosis include the pulmonary infiltrate, enlarged hilar nodes, and lymphangitic streaks which may be seen extending from the enlarged hilar nodes to the pulmonary infiltrate. This is termed "the primary complex." Although reinfection tuberculosis in adults affects mainly the upper lobes, primary tuberculosis may affect any lobe.

The diagnosis is established on the basis of a positive tuberculin test, the chest radiograph, and hopefully, bacteriologic confirmation.

Although in most children the pulmonary lesion of primary tuberculosis will heal spontaneously, in a few cases miliary tuberculosis, pleural effusion, and most importantly, meningitis will develop. This is the most common cause of death in children with pulmonary tuberculosis.

Abednego's condition was recognized promptly as pulmonary tuberculosis and treatment was begun. Unfortunately, the home situation was very bad, a "diagnosis" you established when you saw the two shotgun pellets, one in the back and one in the abdomen. The circumstances surrounding this injury were not clear, but it was known that several months after these radiographs were made, the child fired a revolver at his mother. The child was removed to another state by the family and no follow-up was possible.

OTHER PITFALLS TO AVOID

Decide which statements are true:

This 2 year old boy (Fig. 19) has
- A. Pneumonia
- B. Cardiomegaly
- C. Both of the above
- D. None of the above
- E. Can't tell

FIG. 19

This 2 year old boy (Fig. 20) has
- A. Pneumonia
- B. Cardiomegaly
- C. Is the same patient shown in Figure 19.

FIG. 20

ANSWERS

If you said Figure 19 demonstrated cardiomegaly and pneumonia, you failed to take into account the phase of respiration. There are seven posterior ribs seen on the right side at the level of the diaphragm. This has resulted in crowding of the bronchovascular shadows in the lower lobes, creating the appearance of pneumonia. Note also that the heart has a more transverse lie than in Figure 20. This is also a reflection of the poor inspiration and resulting high diaphragm.

In Figure 20 there are nine posterior ribs seen at the level of the right hemidiaphragm. The lungs are clear and the heart appears normal. This radiograph was made during inspiration just a few seconds after the previous radiograph on the same patient.

Before you evaluate a child for cardiomegaly, pneumonia or even congestive failure you must insist that the level of the right hemidiaphragm be at the ninth or tenth posterior rib in order to be certain that he has taken an adequate inspiration.

FIG. 21

CLASSIC MISTAKES

This child's heart is enlarged (Fig. 21).
  A. True
  B. False
  C. This is a stupid question.
  ANSWER: C.

You can't accurately determine cardiac size from an expiratory radiograph. The level of the right hemidiaphragm is at the seventh posterior rib.

An adequate inspiratory radiograph (Fig. 22) shows clearly that the heart is normal in size. If the level of the diaphragm is between the ninth and tenth posterior ribs, the inspiratory effort is adequate, and the heart size can be evaluated.

In time you will count ribs only occasionally because your brain will have learned to judge lung volume without this step.

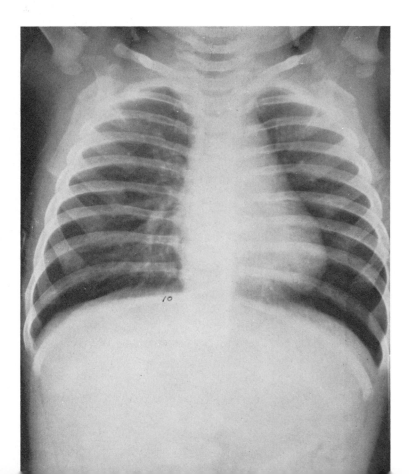

FIG. 22

...AND TIME-HONORED ERRORS

This baby has significant shift of the mediastinum accompanied by a difference in radiodensity of the right and left lungs (Fig. 23).

A. True

B. False

C. This is like the question on the opposite page; it's stupid.

ANSWER: C.

This baby is rotated toward his right, creating the appearance of a mediastinal shift and differential aeration of the lungs. Figure 24 is a straight radiograph, and all is well with the world. No mediastinal shift and normal-appearing lungs. So how can you tell if a radiograph is rotated? You look at the clavicles to see if they are symmetrical, and you look at the anterior ribs to determine whether you can see as much of the anterior ribs on one side as on the other.

(On the right side there are pleural and rib changes caused by previous surgery for tetralogy of Fallot.)

FIG. 23

FIG. 24

IS HIS HEART IN THE RIGHT PLACE?

Jay M., 1 month old, is a "funny looking kid," in that he has a small head with eyes that appear to slant upward and outward, eyelids with thick epicanthal folds, a thickened tongue, separation of the first and second toes, a single deep transverse crease across the palm, and a heart murmur. Also, his heart sounds are heard better in the right hemithorax.

FIGURE 25.   Jay M.

David S. is a 1 month old boy who was examined at a well baby clinic where he appeared to be completely healthy (except for a mild diaper rash). The pediatrician had felt a mass in the left upper quadrant of the abdomen.

FIGURE 26.   David S.

ANSWERS

David S. and *Jay M.* both have dextrocardia. This means that the cardiac apex points to the right (the main muscle mass of the heart is to the right of the spine).

In *David S.'s* case, there is also situs inversus of the abdominal viscera, meaning that the patient's stomach is on his right side and the liver is on the left side (the "mass" felt by the peditrician was, of course, the liver).

Jay M., on the other hand, has his liver on the right side and the stomach on the left side, where they ought to be. This is termed situs solitus, the position of the abdominal organs being normal.

The term applied to *David S.'s* condition is mirror-image dextrocardia. Additional cardiac malformations are rarely encountered. No such abnormality was found in *David*, whose growth and development has been unremarkable.

Jay M. has "situs solitus with dextrocardia." This situation is usually associated with complex congenital heart disease, and it is rarely possible to make a precise anatomic diagnosis without cardiac catheterization. *Jay*, in fact, is a mongoloid; that is, he has Down's syndrome, or trisomy 21. This condition is often associated with an "endocardial cushion defect." This term refers to the four centers of growth from which parts of the mitral and tricuspid valves as well as the contiguous portions of the atrial and ventricular septa are formed. A defect in the endocardial cushions leads to a left-to-right shunt.

Although *Jay* has an endocardial cushion defect, it is more common for patients with situs solitus and dextrocardia to have "corrected transposition of the great vessels," ventricular septal defect with pulmonary stenosis, tricuspid atresia, or other malformations. In other words, usually you can't predict the congenital heart disease in patients with situs solitus and dextrocardia.

A TWO YEAR OLD WITH HYPERTENSION

FIG. 27

Michael B. is a 2 year old boy who appeared to his parents to be in perfect health. However, during a routine physical examination his pediatrician found the blood pressure in the arms to be 140/90, while the blood pressure in the legs was unobtainable. The femoral pulses were present but diminished.

The examination of the chest revealed that the point of maximal impulse was in the fourth intercostal space at the midclavicular line. A grade ii/iv midsystolic murmur was heard.

The AP chest radiograph is presented here (Fig. 27).

ANSWER

Michael's physicians agreed that clinically he had a coarctation of the aorta. They consulted with the surgeons and radiologists and felt that aortography was indicated to define the extent and site of the coarctation. (Aortography is often not necessary since the site of narrowing may be seen on the films and especially during careful fluoroscopy.) Figure 28 is one "cut" from the aortogram. The catheter can be seen entering the aortic arch from the right subclavian artery.

There is a localized constriction in the descending thoracic aorta inferior to the site at which the ductus would be seen if it were patent and opacified. This is termed "adult" or post-ductal coarctation, as opposed to pre-ductal or "infantile" coarctation. In post-ductal coarctation there is a 25 per cent incidence of bicuspid aortic valve, which *Michael* had. (This is significant because of the incidence of subacute bacterial endocarditis upon bicuspid aortic valves.)

Examination of the extensive collateral circulation in this coarctation of the aorta reveals strikingly dilated and tortuous vessels, including the internal mammary arteries and the thyrocervical trunks. Fortunately, there is communication between the collateral circulation above the level of the coarctation and that which is beneath the coarctation, thereby assuring an adequate supply of blood to the lower part of the body despite the reduced blood flow in the aorta.

Why did *Michael* have hypertension? One theory is that the constriction of the aorta causes hypertension on a renal basis, rather like a Goldblatt kidney preparation. Another hypothesis suggests that the hypertension is caused by mechanical factors. There is increased resistance and reduced distensibility of the aorta above the constriction, which may well explain the hypertension in the arms. Actually, both factors may be significant.

The plain films of the chest usually show only a mild cardiomegaly. Rib

FIG. 28

notching, caused by erosion of the ribs due to the enlarged intercostal arteries, is rarely seen under the age of 5 and is barely detectible here. Occasionally the ascending aorta may be prominent, and if a barium swallow is done, there may be a projection on the contour of the barium-opacified esophagus at the site of the coarctation.

When *Michael* was 7 years old he was operated upon and the coarcted segment was removed. An end-to-end anastomosis of the remaining thoracic aorta was performed. The reason that the child was not operated upon at the time of diagnosis was that there was some concern that the region of the anastomosis might not grow. It is preferable to wait until the child and aorta are bigger. Of course, if the child shows early evidence of congestive heart failure, the procedure may be performed when the child is younger.

A SEVEN YEAR OLD WITH CYANOSIS

FIG. 29

Billy G., now 10 years old, was noted at birth to have a cardiac murmur associated with slight but definite cyanosis. At that time he was admitted to another hospital where a diagnosis of congenital heart disease was made. Treatment with digitalis was begun and continued until age 4. Since then he has done well, with minimal cyanosis and normal growth and development. Recently, however, he has begun to have decreased exercise tolerance and increasing cyanosis. He is now admitted for cardiac catheterization and consideration for surgical correction (Fig. 29).

FIGURE 30. Billy G.

ANSWER

The chest radiograph on *Billy* showed normal arrangement of the abdominal viscera. This is implied by the position of the stomach bubble on the patient's left.

Which side is the aortic arch on? Look carefully at the tracheal air shadow. It is deviated slightly to the left. This tells you that the aortic arch is on the right side, and indeed, you can see a rounded density projected over the right fourth interspace. Also, there is no room for the normal aortic arch to the left of the trachea.

The pulmonary vascularity is about normal. The heart size and shape are also normal.

In summary, the plain AP chest radiograph shows normal abdominal situs, normal size and shape of the heart, normal pulmonary vascularity, and a right-sided aortic arch. Figure 30 is one frame of an angiogram which confirms the presence of the right aortic arch. How was the injection made? Are there more findings on the angiogram? What's the diagnosis?

FIGURE 31. Billy G.

FIGURE 32. Billy G.

ANSWER (Cont'd.)

The analysis of any angiogram begins with the catheter position which is seen in Figure 31 with a radiopaque marker on its tip. The lateral view (Fig. 32) shows the right ventricle positioned anteriorly, receiving the injection of contrast material.

The infundibulum is the part of the right ventricular outflow tract just superior to the catheter tip. The tight stenosis seen in both the AP and lateral views is characteristic of this form of congenital heart disease. Sometimes pulmonary valvar stenosis occurs in addition to the infundibular stenosis (and, rarely, there may be total absence of the pulmonary valve).

Figure 30 shows simultaneous opacification of the aorta and pulmonary artery which occurs because of a ventricular septal defect that permits contrast material and blood to flow from the right ventricle to the left ventricle. In Figure 30 you can barely see the infundibular stenosis.

Billy has tetralogy of Fallot. About one-fourth of these patients will have a right-sided aortic arch. Other features of this condition include stenosis of the right ventricular outflow tract, usually at the infundibular level but sometimes at the valvar level or at both levels. This results in right ventricular hypertrophy.

There is also a ventricular septal defect, and the aorta overrides both ventricular cavities. These features are, of course, present but are not demonstrated on this study.

Infants with tetralogy of Fallot are usually initially treated medically until they are older and bigger and are better able to tolerate surgery. Small, frequent feedings and oxygen and morphine for the "blue spells" are important. Nonetheless, some infants will have "blue spells" so often that surgery is mandatory. Direct anastomosis of the aorta to the pulmonary artery will supply more blood to the lungs and can be performed in infancy.

The Blalock-Taussig operation is better suited for older children. In this procedure the subclavian artery is anastomosed to the main branch of the pulmonary artery.

Billy had a "total correction" procedure. This consists of closure of the ventricular septal defect, resection of the infundibular stenosis (or enlarging the volume of the infundibulum with a pericardial patch), and relief of any pulmonic valvar stenosis via valvulotomy. This child has done well clinically since surgery and is now an active child who is gaining weight and growing normally.

A TWO YEAR OLD WITH CYANOSIS

FIGURE 33. Philip G.

Philip G. is a 2 year old boy with cough, fever, and cyanosis who is brought to the Emergency Room by the baby sitter because of his obvious ill appearance. The parents are on vacation, but the baby sitter thinks the child has been seen before at this hospital. A chest x-ray is requested while the record room looks for the old chart.

The x-ray requisition states, "R/O pneumonia." (Further clinical data would have been a help!) How would you report this chest AP and lateral (Figs. 33 and 34)?

FIGURE 34. Philip G.

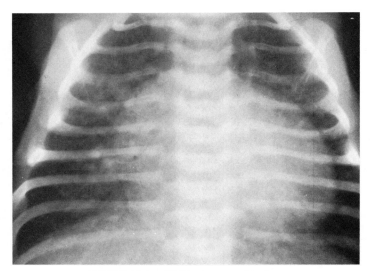

FIGURE 35.   Philip at age 13 days

FIGURE 36.   Philip G.

ANSWER

Philip clearly has a triangular-shaped density superimposed on the left cardiac silhouette; this density represents a collapsed left lower lobe.

The heart appears enlarged and the right fourth and fifth ribs look different from the other ribs. A rib that appears different from its brothers may simply be reflecting the footprints of the cardiac surgeon. Certainly a large heart and rib changes would be consistent with some form of surgically treated congenital heart disease, and usually old films prior to surgery are helpful in establishing the radiologic diagnosis. In *Philip's* case, the file room came up with the master folder; Figure 35 shows *Philip* at age 13 days.

The base of the heart ("vascular pedicle") is very narrow and the pulmonary vascularity is definitely increased. The triad of a cyanotic patient whose chest radiograph shows increased vascularity and a narrow vascular pedicle should suggest the diagnosis which is confirmed on the lateral view of the venous angiogram (Fig. 36). Contrast material is seen in the superior vena cava entering the heart, but note that the aorta is anterior to the pulmonary artery. In case you don't recall, this is abnormal; the normal situation consists of the pulmonary artery anterior to the aorta as seen on the lateral view. Because the great arteries are reversed in location it can be stated that *Philip* has transposition of the great arteries. The aorta rises from the right ventricle and the pulmonary artery rises from the left ventricle. This situation is not compatible with life (think about it!) unless there is mixing of the blood via a shunt such as an atrial septal defect, ventricular septal defect, or patent ductus arteriosus.

Philip had a ventricular septal defect, but to increase the mixing a Rashkind procedure had been performed during the first weeks of his life. This procedure consists of enlarging the patent foramen ovale by pulling a balloon-tipped catheter back through it during cardiac catheterization. This is a temporary measure intended to create enough mixing of blood so that the child can survive until he is old enough for corrective surgery.

The rib change is indeed evidence that open heart surgery was performed, in this case a Blalock-Hanlon procedure. This is the creation of a permanent interatrial communication intended to further improve mixing of blood. (This information was gained by reading the x-ray reports from the film master file. Sometimes if the patient's chart is missing, you can learn a great deal about the patient's prior history from the x-ray reports in the master file.)

At this point we know that *Philip* has transposition of the great vessels treated with a Rashkind procedure and Blalock-Hanlon operation. He has "overcirculation" in the pulmonary circuit (remember the increase in pulmonary vascularity), resulting in an increase in the size of the left atrium. When the left atrium is exceedingly enlarged in infants, it compresses the left lower lobe bronchus, causing atelectasis. (Others think that the collapse is due to the enlarged heart.) Obviously this is difficult to treat, and a series of old films all showed a loss of volume of the left lower lobe to a greater or lesser degree.

Why is the "vascular pedicle" narrowed in Figure 35? With transposition of the great arteries, the ascending aorta is displaced, so that in the frontal projection it superposes the descending aorta. Moreover, the thymus is atrophic. By the way, did you notice that the aorta is narrowed distal to the branching of the great vessels (Fig. 36)? If not, you missed a coarctation of the aorta.

COUGH, FEVER, AND RAPID RESPIRATION AND PULSE IN A THREE MONTH OLD BOY

7-29

FIGURE 37. Kenneth

On July 29, **Kenneth M.** was brought to the Outpatient Clinic by his mother who stated that *Kenneth* was irritable, cried a lot, and had a temperature of 103° rectally. He also coughed so much that he couldn't sleep.

The physical examination confirmed the elevation of the temperature and showed the pulse to be 130 and rate of respiration to be 50 per minute. Examination of the chest revealed wheezing but no rales.

Chest x-ray on July 29 was negative (Fig. 37). *Kenneth* was treated symptomatically.

He returned on August 21 with a recurrence of the same symptoms. How would you report this chest study (Fig. 38)?

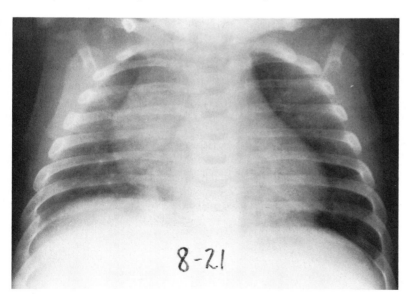

8-21

FIGURE 38. Kenneth M.

ANSWER

The chest radiograph of August 21 has changed; there are two very significant new findings. The early study showed no fluid in the pleural space and no definite consolidation in the lungs. The August 21 film shows obliteration of the right costophrenic sulcus and a small amount of fluid along the right chest wall. This is accompanied by consolidation in a portion of the right lower lobe, close to the heart.

The findings of fluid in the pleural space associated with consolidation in the lung should suggest staphylococcal pneumonia. Usually the radiologist can't predict the bacteriology in a given case (a fact the radiologist *and* clinician frequently forget). However, staphylococcal pneumonia is often an exception. The involvement is unilateral about 80 per cent of the time. The pneumonia is not commonly accompanied by mediastinal lymph node enlargement. Pleural involvement is seen in 90 per cent of the cases, and pneumothorax and pyopneumothorax occur in one-fourth of the cases.

By 11:00 P.M. on August 23, *Kenneth* had formed a small cyst just medial to the gross amount of fluid now present in the right pleural space (Fig. 39). (This baby has been filmed in the supine position.) In most or all instances, a pneumatocele represents a subpleural air collection. Necrosis of a portion of a bronchiolar wall permits air to dissect the interstitial pulmonary tissues, where it forms a tract to the subpleural space. It may occur in a matter of hours, and there may be coalescence of pneumatoceles. It may take months for these cavities to clear.

Is there a differential diagnosis for unilateral consolidation with pleural reaction? Yes; in primary tuberculous pneumonia and, rarely, in pneumococcal pneumonia and *Haemophilus influenzae* pneumonia similar findings may occur. But the additional finding of a pneumatocele is highly suggestive that the causative organism is staphylococcus.

In *Kenneth's* case the diagnosis was suggested by the radiograph. Cultures were taken and treatment initiated on the presumption that this was staphylococcal pneumonia. The cultures of the blood and pleural fluid established that this was correct. The child recovered.

**FIGURE 39.
Kenneth M.**

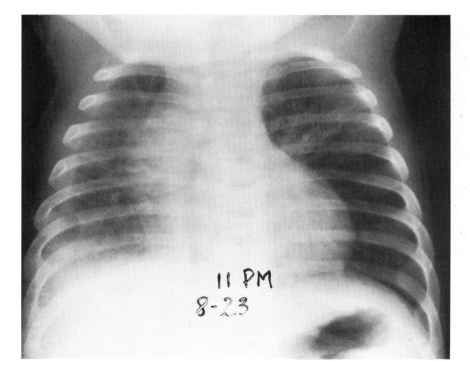

COUGH PRODUCTIVE OF FOUL SPUTUM

FIGURE 40. Debbie E.

FIGURE 41. Debbie E.

Debbie E. is a 12 year old girl who is an old friend of the hospital (she has two hospital charts—both thicker than the Manhattan telephone directory). She returned to the Chest Clinic complaining of producing increasing amounts of foul-smelling sputum associated with decreasing ability to keep up with her friends when they played games that involved any type of exercise.

Debbie is a thin 12 year old, much shorter than her classmates in school. Her chest has a very emphysematous configuration. At examination her vital signs show an increased respiratory rate for her (about 24 per minute) and a temperature of 99.6° orally. Auscultation of the chest reveals bilateral moist rales.

The diagnosis of *Debbie's* chronic condition can be made from the chest PA and lateral views (Figs. 40 and 41), although in *Debbie's* case it was established when she was a baby.

ANSWER

Debbie has cystic fibrosis, a disease of the exocrine glands inherited as an autosomal recessive illness. It involves the pancreas, mucous glands of the bronchi, and salivary and sweat glands. The characteristic secretion of the affected glands is a thick mucus which plugs the ducts.

In the lungs the thick mucus causes occlusion of bronchi and resulting atelectasis. Peribronchial inflammation occurs and the bronchial walls become thickened or "cuffed." Air-trapping occurs and is manifest clinically and radiologically as overinflation. There is a wide AP diameter to the chest, as seen on the lateral view. This is accompanied by the low level of the diaphragm, causing the heart to appear small.

The occlusion of exocrine glands in the pancreas causes atrophy of the parenchyma and results in reduced enzyme secretion and malabsorption. In the newborn, the meconium may be so thick that bowel obstruction occurs. If the meconium leaks into the peritoneal cavity, there is prompt calcification, indicating meconium peritonitis. Obstruction of the bile ducts may lead to biliary cirrhosis, and these children may have gastrointestinal bleeding from esophageal varices.

Other associated conditions include nasal polyps which fill the nasal cavity. Sometimes rectal prolapse occurs.

In *Debbie's* case the pulmonary manifestations are not yet disabling. She has frequent respiratory infections, but appropriate antibiotics and "respiratory toilet" (postural drainage and chest thumping to mobilize secretions) enable her to handle the infections fairly well. The other manifestations of cystic fibrosis do not appear to have affected her clinically.

The diagnosis of cystic fibrosis in children can usually be suspected if emphysema, chronic lung changes, and peribronchial cuffing (better illustrated in a later case) are present together on the radiograph.

FIGURE 42.   Lucifer

THREE NEWBORNS WITH RESPIRATORY DISTRESS

Baby Boy Lucifer (Fig. 42) is a 1900-gram premature newborn who developed rapid respiration, grunting, and retraction of the intercostal spaces approximately one-half hour after birth.

Baby Boy Mephistopheles (Fig. 43) is also premature. This radiograph was taken at 9 hours of age shortly after intubation, which was done because of increasing respiratory distress and cyanosis.

FIGURE 43.   Mephistopheles

FIGURE 44.   Beelzebub

Baby Boy Beelzebub (Fig. 44) was 2 weeks old at the time this radiograph was obtained. He appeared normal for the first seven days and then developed difficulty in breathing while nursing. The physical examination showed that the cardiac apex was shifted to the right, and gurgling sounds were heard on the left side of the chest.

FIGURE 44A. **Normal newborn lungs for comparison**

ANSWERS

Baby Boy Lucifer and *Baby Boy Mephistopheles* both have lungs which are not normally ventilated and which have a reticulonodular, almost granular appearance. If you look closely at *Baby Boy Lucifer's* radiograph there are radiolucent strips which radiate from the hila (air bronchogram). The generic term applied to these lungs is "under-ventilated," or "atelectatic." Many of the alveoli are collapsed; in severe cases, almost all the alveoli are airless. The bronchioles, alveolar ducts, and occasional alveoli are overdistended.

These babies have severe hyaline membrane disease. This condition is usually seen only in premature babies. Clinically, shortly after birth they develop tachypnea, grunting, retraction of the intercostal spaces, and cyanosis.

The pathologic basis for the radiographic features are the "hyaline membranes," which are largely composed of fibrin and are derived from the blood in the infant's pulmonary capillaries. The fibrin deposits cause a decrease in lung compliance and respiratory distress results.

The widespread atelectasis is caused by an absence of surfactant. This substance increases the surface tension in the alveoli; without it the alveoli collapse on expiration. The granular (or reticulonodular) appearance of the lungs is caused by discrete areas of hyperinflation surrounded by atelectatic foci. This also causes the "air bronchogram" effect.

Complications of this condition include pneumothorax and pneumomediastinum.

These babies were treated with oxygen and were given supportive care but did not survive.

FIGURE 45. Beelzebub

Baby Boy Beelzebub's radiograph (Fig. 44) shows peculiar gas-containing structures superimposed on the lungs. As a matter of fact, little bowel gas is seen in the abdomen. This should lead you to suspect that the bowel contents have herniated into the chest and that these structures are dilated gas-filled loops of intestine. You had already suspected this because physical examination revealed gurgling sounds in the child's chest.

Figure 45 shows the barium study performed to prove the diagnosis. This is an older case; today this would not have been done because the plain films establish the diagnosis.

This patient had a **diaphragmatic hernia** through the foramen of Bochdalek.

This is due to persistence of one of the pleuroperitoneal canals. It usually occurs on the left side (maybe because the liver inhibits its occurrence on the right side). The hernia may involve the liver, kidney, spleen, the stomach, small bowel, or colon.

Immediately after the diagnosis was made, surgery was performed, and the abdominal contents were replaced. Sometimes there will be compression of the lung on the side opposite the diaphragmatic hernia and that lung will fail to expand. That was not the case with *Baby Boy Beelzebub* and he had an uncomplicated recovery.

(By the way, did you notice that the "Normal newborn" (Fig. 44 A) has a fractured left clavicle?)

ABDOMEN

THREE PATIENTS WITH FEVER AND ABDOMINAL PAIN

FIGURE 46. Trelawney Hope

Trelawney Hope, age 12, the great grandson of the Right Honorable Trelawney Hope was visiting the United States with his rock group called the "Stones" (he plays the electric harmonica) when he became ill. Initially he developed vague abdominal pain and nausea which he attributed to a change in diet. After several hours he began to vomit, and the pain migrated to the right lower quadrant of the abdomen. The manager of the rock group took the boy to the emergency room of the nearest hospital.

Physical examination confirmed tenderness in the right lower quadrant of the abdomen. A rectal examination suggested a mass in the same region.

T 99.8° (orally), P 100, R 16, WBC 9000— normal differential.

Have you seen these names somewhere before?

Mlle. H. Fournaye, age 11, also a member of the "Stones" had exactly the same symptoms as *Trelawney Hope.* There was no abdominal tenderness and definitely no signs of peritoneal irritation. The only positive physical findings were reduced hearing (probably nerve deafness, an occupational hazard) and dullness to percussion with bronchial breath sounds in the right lower lobe area.

T 103° (orally), P 120, R 28, WBC 28,000.

FIGURE 47. Mlle. H. Fournaye

Eduardo Lucas of West Indian descent and also a member of the English rock group, the "Stones," had a urinary tract infection. Figure 48 was the preliminary radiograph for an IVP.

FIGURE 48. Eduardo Lucas

ANSWERS

Trelawney Hope's supine view of the abdomen demonstrates curvature of the lumbar spine with convexity toward the left. This curvature is caused by right psoas muscle spasm and suggests an inflammatory process in the area of the right psoas muscle. (Unfortunately, curvature of the spine may be fortuitous in patients who are not carefully positioned on the x-ray table. This observation is more useful if it is present on the supine *and* upright views of the abdomen.)

Carefully look at the right lower quadrant and you will see a calcific density superimposed on the iliac crest. A coned-down view of this area (Fig. 49) showed this to be a "real" observation. This shadow represents a fecalith, indicates appendicitis, and requires surgery.

Other radiologic findings of appendicitis (not seen here) include ileus of the lower small bowel and a soft tissue fullness in the right lower quadrant, indicative of a mass. (This is seen especially in patients with peri-appendiceal abscess.)

At surgery there was a pinpoint perforation in the tip of the appendix around which there was a small abscess containing the fecalith. Recovery was slow because of the perforation, but now *Trelawney* is again blowing the electric harmonica with his rock group. He has subsequently changed the name of his group from the "Stones" to the "Appendicoliths."

FIGURE 49. Trelawney Hope

Mlle. Fournaye's supine view of the abdomen is normal. (Yes, we worried that there might be fecaliths in the right lower quadrant, but a coned-down view of that area showed only small fecal masses and gas in the cecum and ascending colon.)

A patient with abdominal pain requires chest radiographs because lower lobe pneumonia may cause diaphragmatic irritation and referral of pain to the abdomen. Figure 50 shows just that: consolidation in the right lower lobe.

After Gram stain of the sputum and cultures, *Mlle. Fournaye* was started on antibiotic therapy. Her fever remitted promptly and she still possesses her appendix. Unfortunately her hearing continues to deteriorate, but she is proud of this because she feels a common bond with Beethoven.

Eduardo was known to have sickle cell anemia, and one of the manifestations of this disease is gallstone formation. Figure 48 shows two faceted gallstones in the right upper quadrant of the abdomen. Other anemias, including thalassemia and acquired hemolytic anemias, may also be accompanied by gallstone formation.

Some of the other manifestations of sickle cell disease include formation of thrombi in various organs, cardiomegaly, and infarction of bone, brain, lungs, kidney, or spleen. These children are particularly susceptible to Salmonella infection.

In the case of *Eduardo*, the gallstones were an incidental finding on the preliminary film of the IVP which showed clearly that the stones were not in the kidney. He had no symptoms of cholelithiasis, and he has not yet had a cholecystectomy. His fever and abdominal pain were secondary to his urinary tract infection.

FIGURE 50. Mlle. Fournaye

AND TWO MORE CHILDREN WITH ABDOMINAL PAIN

Percy Trevelyan, a 3 year old boy, was feeling completely well, according to his mother, when he suddenly developed abdominal pain. The boy subsequently passed a bloody stool which alarmed Mrs. Trevelyan and caused her to bring the boy to the hospital.

The physical examination revealed an acutely ill child in obvious pain but with normal vital signs. There was a mass in the right lower quadrant of the abdomen that was soft and only minimally tender. There was no rigidity or rebound tenderness. Otherwise the abdominal examination was negative. The pediatrician put the clinical history together with the physical findings and made a tentative diagnosis. He sent the boy to the radiology department for confirmation *and* treatment.

FIGURE 51. Percy Trevelyan

A 13 year old girl, **Miss Blessington,** appeared one afternoon in the Emergency Room complaining of urgency and frequent urination accompanied by pain in the suprapubic region. She had been seen in the Child Psychiatry Clinic because of a behavior disorder and the intern wondered if her symptoms weren't simply a part of her pattern of behavior.

The physical examination was negative, but a urinalysis showed WBC's and bacteria TNTC (too numerous to count). An IVP was requested and Figure 52 is part of the preliminary plain film of the abdomen. After seeing this film the intern requested a urology consultation, suspecting that this child had bladder stones. The radiologist questioned the child and took another radiograph which proved the diagnosis. What question did he ask *Miss Blessington* and what radiograph did he obtain?

FIGURE 52. Miss Blessington

FIGURE 53. Percy Trevelyan

ANSWERS

Percy's radiologic workup was begun with a supine view of the abdomen (Fig. 51). This showed a soft tissue density in the right lower quadrant of the abdomen consistent with an ileocolic intussusception. In this condition, the proximal bowel telescopes into the distal bowel. It may sometimes be caused by a polyp or Meckel's diverticulum, but often no cause is found for the intussusception.

Initial treatment consists of confirmation of the diagnosis and hydrostatic reduction of the intussusception by means of barium enema. Care is taken to ensure that no pressure is exerted on the abdomen or the barium bag, and that the enema tube is not "milked." The barium bag is adjusted to a height of 2½ feet above the x-ray table. A "spot film" (Fig. 53) shows the "coiled spring" appearance which is characteristic of intussusception.

Reduction is considered to be complete when there is free flow of barium into the small bowel from a normally filled cecum. If this can't be demonstrated, surgical reduction will be necessary; however, in about two-thirds to three fourths of the cases of intussusception, the barium enema will be both diagnostic and therapeutic.

Percy also has cystic fibrosis which you can recognize from the chest film (Fig. 54) and from the edge of the abdominal film (Fig. 51) because of the peribronchial cuffing seen well overlying the right fourth rib posteriorly and left fifth rib posteriorly. Changes are also visible in the lung bases in Figure 51. Cystic fibrosis is a known, but not common, cause of intussusception. In *Percy's* case, the intussusception could not be reduced with a barium enema and surgery was necessary.

FIGURE 54.   Percy Trevelyan

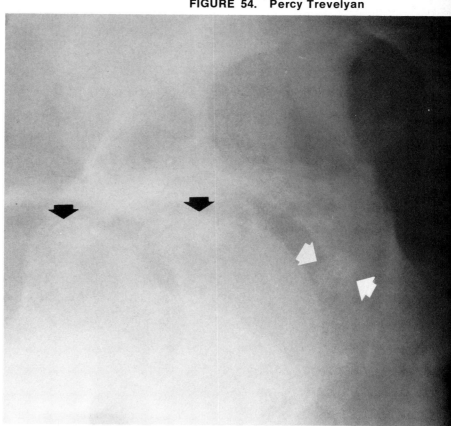

FIGURE 55.   Miss Blessington

Bladder stones are very rare in children in the absence of a neurogenic bladder or severe chronic infection. The radiologist obtained a lateral view (Fig. 55) which showed the densities to be posterior and in the rectum (white arrows). The black arrows indicate the not-quite-superimposed femoral heads. He then questioned *Miss Blessington* and learned that she had been receiving iron tablets for the treatment of excessive menstrual bleeding. She

showed him the tablets, and they corresponded in size and shape to the densities seen in Figure 52.

It turned out that the child also had cystitis and this accounted for her symptoms and urinalysis findings. An IVP was not performed. A common but not universal rule is that a structural cause for infection should be sought after the second urinary tract infection in a girl and after the first urinary tract infection in a boy.

TWO BABIES WITH VOMITING AND DEHYDRATION

FIGURE 56. Alec Cunningham

Alec Cunningham, 3 weeks old, developed projectile vomiting (this means that the vomitus clears the chin and distinguishes it from drooling) during the second week of life. His abdomen became distended, and peristaltic waves were clearly visible through the abdominal wall.

When first seen at the hospital this boy was dehydrated. Examination of the abdomen suggested a tumor mass, the size of an olive, in the region of the outlet of the stomach.

The surgical resident was sufficiently uncertain of the diagnosis to request an upper G.I. series to confirm his impression (Fig. 56). (The collection of barium above the body of the stomach is in the fourth portion of the duodenum behind the stomach and is not in an ulcer crater.)

Baron Maupertuis, a 7 month old boy, was brought to his pediatrician because of bile-stained vomitus. He had had intermittent abdominal pains and vomiting before, and now his mother was alarmed by the return of his symptoms.

The *Baron* appeared ill and weighed only 9 lbs. 14 oz. (an increase of only 2 lbs. 14 oz. since birth). His vital signs were normal, but the child was mildly dehydrated. His abdomen was tender, but there were no signs of peritoneal irritation.

The *Baron* was admitted to the hospital and an upper G.I. series was performed (Fig. 57).

FIGURE 57. Baron Maupertuis

FIGURE 58. Alec Cunningham

ANSWERS

The striking feature of *Alec Cunningham's* upper G.I. series is the extreme length of the pyloric channel. Figure 58 is a "spot film" that also demonstrates its narrowness. The ribbon-like strips of barium extending from the antrum to the duodenal bulb are explained by the fact that the pyloric canal is not a circular tube; instead, the mucosa has many longitudinal folds in which the barium is trapped. When radiographed, as in Figure 58, the barium in the canal therefore has a ribbon-like or railroad track appearance.

This, then, is hypertrophic pyloric stenosis. It is much more common in males than females and usually begins several weeks after birth. In this condition the circular pyloric muscle is hypertrophied, with secondary narrowing of the pyloric canal and redundancy of the mucosa.

The etiology is unknown, but there is a distinct familial tendency. The diagnosis is established upon palpation of the "pyloric olive." Only rarely, perhaps in 1 case in 10, will an upper G.I. series be necessary, and only then because the history is confusing or the physical examination equivocal.

In the past, medical management (antispasmodics and thickened feedings) was used to treat hypertrophic pyloric stenosis. Today, the Ramstedt pyloromyotomy is the treatment of choice. In this operation a lengthwise incision is made through the hypertrophied pyloric muscle, and the mucosa is allowed to prolapse through the incised area. This relieves the gastric outlet obstruction and almost invariably the symptoms promptly disappear.

The *Baron's* upper G.I. series and the coned-down view of the duodenum show an abnormal position of the third and fourth portions of the duodenum and of the duodenal-jejunal junction. The third portion should pass horizontally from the right to the left of the spine, and the fourth portion should ascend, so that the duodenal-jejunal junction is at the same height as the junction of the first and second portions of the duodenum. In the *Baron*, duodenal-jejunal junction is displaced downward and to the right of the spine. The malposition of the distal one-half of the duodenum is the tip-off that the Baron has intestinal malrotation.

The fetal gastrointestinal tract is a straight tube initially. At the fifth week of fetal life the midgut (which comprises the distal duodenum, the small bowel, and about the proximal one-half of the colon) elongates and soon herniates into what will become the umbilical cord. At the same time, the cecum moves to the patient's left and the duodenum-jejunum to the patient's right, as rotation of the midgut begins. The duodenum and the colon are close together at this point. If rotation arrests at this stage of development, or at any subsequent stage before the duodenal-jejunal junction is in the normal location, bands frequently form between the duodenum and colon. Also, the attachment of the small bowel mesentery about the origin of the superior mesenteric artery is abnormal and predisposes to midgut volvulus with the superior mesenteric artery as the axis for the twist.

The *Baron* has one of the two complications of malrotation. The bands, frequently referred to as Ladd's bands, extend from the right colon across the duodenum to the upper abdomen and cause intermittent extrinsic compres-

FIGURE 59. Baron Maupertuis

sion of the duodenum, obstruction and bilious vomiting.

The second complication of malrotation is volvulus of the midgut about the superior mesenteric artery. This is allowed by the incomplete fixation of the small bowel mesentery and may result in infarction of the midgut. A third and rarer complication is chronic malabsorption.

About one-half of the patients with malrotation will be seen in the first week of life. The remaining cases are present throughout childhood and sometimes into adulthood.

The *Baron* had surgical correction of the malrotation. The "Ladd's bands" compressing the duodenum were divided. The intestine was inspected; volvulus had not developed. Then the intestines were returned to the abdominal cavity and the ascending colon was fixed on the left side and the duodenum-jejunum was fixed on the right side. This position has been found to prevent volvulus later on.

TWO CHILDREN WITH ABDOMINAL CRAMPS AND DIARRHEA

FIGURE 60. Willy

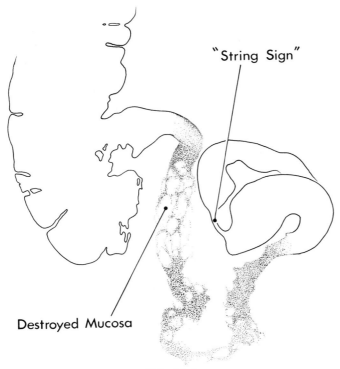

"String Sign"

Destroyed Mucosa

FIG. 60 A

Willy (full name: **Wilhelm Gottsreich Sigismond von Ormstein,** Grand Duke of Cassel-Falstein and hereditary King of Bohemia), age 14, had a history of several years of cramping abdominal pain associated with fever and diarrhea. The diarrhea was accompanied by excessive mucus in the stools and, rarely, blood. His weight gain had been slow, and he appeared chronically ill.

Physical examination revealed a small boy, slender and somewhat cachectic. The oral temperature was 99.6°, but the other vital signs were normal. The pertinent physical findings included tenderness in the right lower quadrant, where there was an ill-defined mass. There were no rectal fistulas. A barium enema was performed at which time reflux occurred into the terminal ileum (Fig. 60).

FIGURE 61. Clotilde Lothman

Clotilde Lothman (full name: **von Saxe-Meningen,** second daughter of the king of Scandinavia), age 16, was incapacitated by bloody diarrhea occurring about 15 times daily. The feces were watery and contained pus and mucus as well as blood. The diarrhea was accompanied by cramping abdominal pain.

Physical examination showed a chronically ill child. She had had iritis and arthritis ˙ɹ the past.

Her abdomen was diffusely tender but no mass could be palpated. There was also no evidence of peritoneal irritation or of cutaneous fistulas. The radiographs presented here are the AP and left anterior oblique views of the abdomen obtained during barium enema examination (Figs. 61 and 62).

FIGURE 62. Clotilde Lothman

ANSWERS

The radiologist doing *Willy's* barium enema has used a pressure paddle with a metallic rim to separate the loops of terminal ileum. In the center of the field encompassed by the pressure paddle there is an area of ileum in which the intestinal lumen shows irregular coating with barium and destruction of the normal mucosal pattern. The more proximal ileum appears normal except for a short involved area. The "skipping" of areas of involvement is typical of this condition, as is the markedly narrowed lumen seen best in the proximal area of involvement. Because the lumen is no wider than a string, this has been termed the "string sign."

At fluoroscopy, the radiologist looked for fistulas and for involvement of the cecum. The right lower quadrant of the abdomen was quite tender during palpation with the pressure paddle, but colonic involvement and fistulas were not found.

Willy has regional enteritis (Crohn's disease). This condition characteristically involves discrete segments of the small bowel. Initially the bowel wall is thickened and becomes stenosed and fibrotic in the late stages of the disease. The process is accompanied by apparent obstruction of the lymphatics and thickening of the mesentery. Microscopically noncaseating granulomas are seen deep in the bowel wall. Areas of necrosis may occur, and fistulas may form.

The etiology of regional enteritis is unknown. The classic clinical presentation of diarrhea and cramps is not always seen, especially in children. Some children present with growth failure and are found to have a delayed bone age, so that hypopituitarism is suspected. Other children are seen because of rectal fistulas or intestinal obstruction, while still others have symptoms that suggest acute appendicitis. The stomach, duodenum, jejunum, and colon as well as the ileum may be involved, and the symptoms will vary accordingly.

Treatment consists of a low-residue diet and a nonabsorbable sulfonamide, salicylazosulfapyridine (Azulfidine). Steroids have occasionally been used. Surgery is ordinarily reserved for controlling the complications of regional enteritis, such as bowel obstruction, fistulas, and perforation.

Willy continues to exist in symbiosis with his disease, which he regards as a chronic disability. He and his physicians do not think in terms of cure but in terms of long-term control of the symptoms. At the time this is written, the child is able to participate in school, but his grades suffer from frequent absences. His parents are concerned that progression of the disease will eventually restrict his activities and limit his ability to attend school and participate in normal childhood activities.

Clotilde was admitted to the hospital. A barium enema was performed only after preliminary views of the abdomen showed no evidence of "toxic megacolon." (The clinical diagnosis was ulcerative colitis, and if the bowel had become acutely dilated and friable, this condition would have been termed toxic megacolon. In this situation, a barium enema might perforate the colon and spill barium into the peritoneal cavity.) The AP, left anterior oblique, and coned-down views (Fig. 63) of the descending colon show deep and superficial ulcers in the bowel wall. The diameter of the lumen of the descending colon is reduced, and no haustrations are seen.

Clotilde has not only the clinical but also the radiologic findings of ulcerative colitis. The disease ordinarily begins in the rectum or sigmoid colon, which are better evaluated by proctoscopy and sigmoidoscopy than by barium enema.

The mucosa can be inspected through the proctoscope or sigmoidoscope and will be found to bleed easily. Minute ulcers in the mucosa may be detected as well. Later the ulcers may coalesce so that the islands of remaining mucosa appear as pseudopolyps. As the disease progresses, the bowel becomes shortened with "lead pipe rigidity." In children with a history of ulcerative colitis for several years, there is a definite risk of supervening carcinoma of the colon, a complication that may be difficult to recognize radiologically.

The etiology of ulcerative colitis is unknown. It is regarded as a systemic disease because of the frequently associated systemic manifestations, which include iritis, arthritis, erythema nodosum, and *pyoderma gangrenosum.*

The treatment depends upon the stage of the disease and the extent of involvement. Steroids, blood transfusions, and supportive measures are necessary in the acute fulminating phase of the disease. A low-residue diet, Azulfidine, steroids, and sometimes psychiatric care are useful during the chronic indolent phase of ulcerative colitis. Surgery is advised when the patient has perforation of the colon, is exsanguinating from colonic bleeding, has toxic megacolon, or is unresponsive to medical management. Many gastroenterologists and surgeons advise colectomy to eliminate the very substantial risk of carcinoma of the colon.

At this time *Clotilde* is being managed medically. She seems to be doing only fairly well, and her parents have been informed of the risk of carcinoma, and we suspect that they will agree to total colectomy in the near future.

FIGURE 63. Clotilde, spot film

TWO NEWBORN BABIES WITH FEEDING DIFFICULTY

FIGURE 64.   Neville

Baby Boy Neville St. Clair, 2 days old, was the product of a normal full-term pregnancy. Shortly after birth, his abdomen began to become distended and mucous secretions accumulated about his mouth. He regurgitated his first and only feeding. The pediatric intern was unable to pass a nasogastric tube into the stomach. He made a presumptive diagnosis, and it was confirmed by the radiographs of the chest (Figs. 64 and 65) which were obtained after 1 cc. of contrast material (oily Dionosil) was injected into the esophageal pouch through the tube.

Review of these radiographs established the diagnosis, and treatment was initiated.

FIGURE 65.   Neville

Baby Girl Kate Whitney was the product of a normal pregnancy and delivery. Her physical examination at birth was negative. However, feedings were initiated with great difficulty because each feeding caused coughing, choking, and cyanosis. A chest radiograph in the newborn nursery suggested pneumonia. The radiologist reviewed the history with the pediatricians and suggested an esophagram (Fig. 66).

FIGURE 66. Kate

ANSWERS

Baby Boy Neville St. Clair's radiographs demonstrate that the esophagus is dilated and ends in a blind pouch. The air in the stomach (both views) indicates that there must be a connection between the outside atmosphere and the gastrointestinal tract. Since the proximal esophagus is atretic, there must be a distal tracheoesophageal fistula. This is the most common form of the esophageal atresia–tracheoesophageal fistula complex.

Notice that there are bilateral upper lobe infiltrates. *Neville* was unable to swallow his saliva or his first feeding, resulting in aspiration of both.

Neville was started on antibiotic therapy and then surgery was performed. The distal tracheoesophageal fistula was ligated, and the two esophageal segments were anastomosed.

Had *Neville* been too ill to tolerate a primary anastomosis, a gastrostomy would have been performed for decompression of the gastrointestinal tract and for feeding. Then, when his condition was stable, the definitive surgery would have been performed.

As it was, *Neville* did well following surgery. At the age of 10 months a barium swallow showed minimal narrowing at the level of the anastomosis of the two portions of the esophagus and abnormal peristalsis in the middle third of the esophagus.

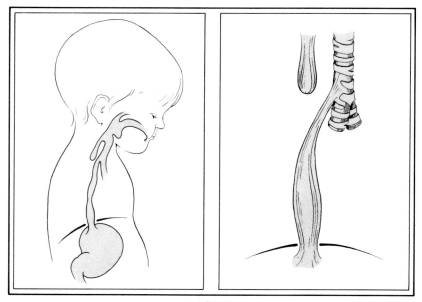

FIG. 67

(Redrawn from *The Surgery of Infancy and Childhood,* with permission of Dr. Robert Gross)

When *Baby Girl Kate Whitney* was seen by her pediatrician, it was not clear whether she was aspirating her feedings because of incoordinated swallowing or had a tracheoesophageal fistula. (Esophageal atresia had been ruled out by passing a nasogastric tube into the stomach.) A contrast study (Fig. 66) demonstrated a fistulous communication low in the neck, between the trachea and esophagus. (Barium was not used because the radiologist was afraid that if it was aspirated or there was a "T–E" fistula, barium might enter the lungs. Oily Dionisil was used—the same agent used for bronchograms.)

Kate has an isolated tracheoesophageal fistula. The fistula was ligated and divided. Recovery was prompt, and the child has had no further difficulties.

AN INFANT WITH CONTINUOUS PURULENT DISCHARGE FROM THE LEFT NOSTRIL

John Openshaw was an infant who had a chronic purulent discharge from the left nostril, which seemed to be plugged. The pediatrician suspected that the child had unilateral choanal atresia because he was unable to pass a catheter through the left nostril down to the level of the oropharynx. *John* was referred to the radiology department for a "choanogram."

For this procedure, the patient is placed in the supine position and immobilized by a sheet that is elaborately wrapped around him (mummification); this is really quite comfortable. The radi-

ologist then passed a radiopaque catheter into the right nostril and documented its patency with a lateral radiograph of the nasal and oropharynx (Fig. 68).

A catheter was then introduced into the left nostril where it met total obstruction. The secretions that had accumulated in the nostril were removed and the radiologist tried again, with no success. He then injected 3 cc. of oily Dionosil through the catheter and the technologist obtained three views of the area: a lateral view (Fig. 69), the AP view (Fig. 70), and the base view (Fig. 71).

FIGURE 68. John Openshaw

FIG. 69

ANSWER

John Openshaw's radiographs demonstrated that there is a total obstruction of the left choana (posterior naris). The obstruction is caused by a membranous or bony partition that closes the nasal airway above the posterior end of the hard palate. This condition may be unilateral or bilateral and is known as choanal atresia.

Bilateral choanal atresia is especially serious in the newborn because it may take days for the baby to learn mouth-breathing. Because of the dependency on nasal breathing, the newborn may die of asphyxia if choanal atresia is not recognized. Some babies with bilateral choanal atresia will quickly learn to breathe through the mouth but upon feeding become cyanotic and dyspneic. Unilateral choanal atresia is not as serious a condition in the newborn period. It usually is not recognized until the child is evaluated for unilateral nasal obstruction or abnormal quality of the voice.

Treatment of bilateral choanal atresia is initiated by maintenance of an oral airway. The child may be fed with a stomach tube or medicine dropper until he learns to suck and breathe alternately. If the obstruction is caused by a membrane, it may be resected, utilizing an anterior nasal approach. A bony partition causing obstruction requires a transpalatal approach and removal of the obstruction. The main post-operative problem is restenosis of the posterior choanae.

No definitive surgery is planned at the present time for *John*. The plan is to encourage the mother to keep the nose clean of accumulated secretions, and if the child's voice does not have an abnormal quality, surgery will be delayed until the baby is older, or it may be omitted altogether.

FIG. 70

FIG. 71

TWO NEWBORN BABIES WITH INCREASING ABDOMINAL DISTENTION AND NO STOOLS

Baby Girl Mary Sutherland was less than 12 hours old when her abdomen began to appear distended. At 20 hours she began to vomit greenish material. At the end of her first day no meconium had yet been passed.

The initial physical examination at the time of delivery showed nothing abnormal. The baby was re-examined at 12 hours because the nurses in the newborn nursery were concerned about the abdominal distention. (A smart house officer can learn a lot of pediatrics from the nurses. If communication lines are in good working order, the nurses will inform him of small problems before they become big problems and of big problems before they become disasters.) The house officer found *Baby Girl Sutherland* unchanged since his initial physical examination except that her abdomen was protuberant and the flanks bulged. He could feel no abdominal masses.

The baby was re-examined at 24 hours because of vomiting, lack of stools, and persistent abdominal distention. Included in the workup was a supine view of the chest and abdomen (Fig. 72).

FIGURE 72. Mary Sutherland

Baby Boy Hosmer Angel appeared to be normal at birth. Like *Baby Girl Mary Sutherland*, he developed abdominal distention and passed no meconium during the first day of life. The baby began to appear ill with pallor and increased respiratory rate. A "sepsis workup" (culture of the blood, urine, cerebrospinal fluid, and tracheal aspirate, with Gram stain to help identify any bacteria) was done. An AP view of the abdomen (Fig. 73) was obtained.

The radiologists interpreted this view of the abdomen as showing distended loops of bowel with an especially distended portion of the gut in the right lower quadrant in the region where the cecum would be expected to be. (In babies it is very hard to differentiate small bowel from colon by a plain radiograph. The only way to be certain is to perform a contrast enema.) The radiologists were concerned about a collection of gas bubbles in the right lower quadrant and speculated that this was an abscess. It was suggested that the other areas of bowel were distended on the basis of ileus secondary to obstruction by the abscess. The differential diagnosis included a cecal perforation and appendicitis with periappendiceal abscess, which is rare in newborn full-term infants.

Baby Boy Hosmer was operated upon, and at surgery the cecum was found to be grossly distended. There were two pinpoint perforations from which bowel contents had contaminated the peritoneal cavity near the cecum. A cecostomy was done to decompress the cecum, and the baby was treated with antibiotics.

It is very rare for a newborn baby to "blow out" the cecum, but when it occurs a second associated diagnosis should come to mind. What further measures should be taken?

FIGURE 73.
Hosmer Angel

ANSWERS

The pediatric house officer caring for *Baby Girl Sutherland* did not believe the report of free air in the peritoneal cavity that was called to him in the newborn nursery from the radiology department. So, he descended to the subterranean depths of the hospital to the pediatric radiology department and reviewed the radiographs with the pediatric radiologists. It was pointed out that the linear shadow projected over the right side of the lower thoracic vertebral bodies was the falciform ligament. This extends from the diaphragm and anterior abdominal wall to the caudal edge of the liver and, being water dense, can't be seen unless outlined by air. Furthermore, the large mass of air in the peritoneal cavity forms an oval shape on the supine radiograph as it outlines the edge of the peritoneal cavity (Fig. 72).

To expedite the surgery and to convince the skeptical, an upright abdominal radiograph was taken which again showed the falciform ligament (Fig. 74, arrow). In addition, the spleen and liver have fallen away from the diaphragm, and the superior portion of the peritoneal cavity is filled with air.

At surgery, an ileal stenosis with perforation was found; this was resected, and an end-to-end anastomosis was performed. The etiology of the stenosis was not determined, but the possibility of an intrauterine bowel infarction possibly caused by a local volvulus was raised. *Baby Girl Sutherland* recovered promptly from her surgery and has subsequently gone home and seems well on return visits to the Outpatient Department.

FIGURE 74. Mary Sutherland

Baby Boy Hosmer Angel, soon regained his birth weight. His cecostomy functioned well, and he seemed to thrive in the nursery.

It is well known that in adults an obstruction in the colon, either inflammatory or neoplastic, may present clinically as cecal perforation. Diverticulitis and carcinoma of the colon don't occur in the newborn, but another condition does and the workup for this includes a barium enema (Figs. 75 and 76).

The lateral projection (Fig. 75) demonstrates a contracted segment of lower sigmoid colon (arrows). Above the site of the narrowing, the colon displays bizarre irregular contractions with a saw-toothed appearance. These are the radiologic findings of Hirschsprung's disease.

In this condition, the parasympathetic innervation of the affected portion of the colon including the ganglion cells is absent. The parasympathetic system is responsible for the propulsive contractility of the colon. When the ganglion cells of the myenteric plexus are absent, a physiologic obstruction occurs with dilation of the bowel proximal to the area of absent ganglion cells. The lateral view of the colon shows this contracted segment. However, ganglion cells are absent from this point distally to the anus. The diagnosis was proved by rectal biopsy which showed absence of the ganglion cells.

The initial treatment for this condition is decompressive colostomy or cecostomy proximal to the aganglionic segment. This diverts the fecal stream and prevents the complication of enterocolitis. The aim of surgery is to reconstitute normal function of the colon. This is performed by removing the functionally obstructing segment of the colon or rerouting the fecal stream so as to anastomose normal colon to the anus.

FIG. 75

FIG. 76

THE CASE OF THE MISSING ANUS

Baby Boy Jabez Wilson was discovered to have entered this world incompletely equipped. In place of an anus he had a small dimple that didn't communicate with the large bowel within, in other words, an imperforate anus. The workup for this included a supine view of the abdomen and chest (Fig. 77). The metallic density is an umbilical cord clamp. The study shows absence of gas in the rectum and a normal lumbar spine and sacrum.

The latter point may help to distinguish the two principal types of imperforate anus: high and low. Spine abnormalities are common with the high anomaly but are infrequent with the low.

In the high anomaly, the rectal pouch ends above the pelvic floor (actually the levator ani muscles). A fistula usually is present, extending from the rectum to the posterior urethra or bladder in boys and to the vagina in girls. This high anomaly is treated initially by a colostomy, followed one to two years later by an exacting

FIGURE 77. Jabez Wilson

FIG. 78

abdominoperineal operation. The fistula is divided and the distal colon is pulled through the pelvic floor, attempting to establish as normal a relationship as possible of the terminal colon to the levator ani sling. Finally the pouch is attached at the anal dimple, and an opening is made.

In the low anomaly the rectum passes normally through the levator ani sling. Repair is simpler and is usually done shortly after birth, using only a perineal approach. When fistulas occur they are to the perineum, the base of the scrotum, or the vestibule.

Practically, the clinical differentiation of high and low anomalies may be made by determining the site of the fistula, if present. Of course, a major concern is the distance between the blind rectal pouch and the anal dimple. The classic way to show this has been an "upside-down view" (Figs. 78 and 79). The theory is that the gas in the colon will seek the highest level. If a marker is placed on the anal dimple and a true lateral view of the pelvis obtained with the baby held upside down, a close approximation of the distance between the blind rectal pouch and the anal dimple may be possible. This was done with *Baby Boy Jabez Wilson* (Fig. 78). At 14 hours after birth there was a 2 cm. separation between the distal bowel gas and anal dimple. Fortunately another radiograph (Fig. 79) taken 22 hours after birth shows the separation to be less than 1 cm. The implication from this second film is that this is a low anomaly and repair *can* be performed using the much simpler perineal approach. Why was the distance greater 14 hours after birth? Presumably the swallowed air had not yet reached the rectum or had not displaced the meconium already there.

Most pediatric radiologists have learned to interpret the upside-down view with caution, since at times it may not accurately reflect the anatomy. A low anomaly may appear to be high, as it did on the 14-hour film of *Baby Boy Wilson*, or a high anomaly may appear to be low if the film is made as the infant strains vigorously. Clinical and radiographic assessment of the site of the fistula more reliably differentiates high and low anomalies.

Jabez Wilson's surgery was successful, and he had had an uneventful childhood.

Any idea of the derivation of the patients' names?

FIG. 79

THE CASE OF THE DOUBLE BUBBLE

Baby Girl Culverton Smith, 4 days old, had had bilious vomiting since birth and was quite dehydrated.

The physical examination did not reveal the cause of the vomiting. A supine AP radiograph of the abdomen (Fig. 80) demonstrated only a small amount of air in the stomach. A nasogastric tube was placed in the stomach and gastric contents were aspirated. Then air was injected into the stomach and supine and upright views were obtained (Figs. 81 and 82). (Did you note the different appearance of the sacrum?)

FIG. 81

FIG. 80

FIG. 82

ANSWER

Air as contrast material is not emphasized as much as the more expensive water-soluble contrast agents (Gastrografin, Renografin) or old reliable barium. Actually, the upright view of the abdomen with air injected into the stomach yields all the information available without the risk of the other materials. (The water-soluble contrast materials should almost never be given by mouth to babies. Because of their hyperosmolarity, water is drawn into the small bowel, and the baby becomes profoundly dehydrated.) Barium may be used, but if the baby vomits, he may have trouble clearing the vomitus from the facial area and may aspirate barium into the lungs. Air in moderate amounts is diagnostic; it is also safe, available, and cheap.

The analysis of the upright radiograph shows two air-fluid interfaces. The one to the left of the spine is in the stomach. Review of the supine abdominal view shows air in the stomach and duodenum but not further along in the small bowel. The air-fluid interface to the right of the spine ought to be in the duodenum and there should be an obstruction *distal* to the ampulla of Vater because of the bilious character of the vomitus.

This radiologic pattern is called the "double bubble sign," and it is seen in only a few conditions. At surgery *Culverton Smith* had duodenal atresia, but the "double bubble sign" is also seen in annular pancreas, in which the duodenal obstruction is caused by extrinsic compression. Much more commonly the sign is seen with midgut volvulus. Intrinsic obstruction of the duodenum may also occur if there is severe duodenal stenosis.

The differentiation of the several possibilities mentioned above can be aided by looking at the corners of the radiograph. For example, it is known that duodenal atresia is associated with mongolism. If the pelvis shows flared iliac wings and flattened acetabular roofs, duodenal atresia should be at the top of the list because the patient is likely to be a mongoloid. (This pelvis does not suggest mongolism.) Likewise, if a barium enema shows a malposition of the cecum, malrotation with midgut volvulus should be diagnosis *numero uno*.

The problem, in fact, is a surgical problem, but the aim of the radiologist is to narrow the possible causes so that the surgeon will have some idea of what to expect and will be able to plan accordingly. The child was successfully operated upon for duodenal atresia.

THREE TEENAGERS: ONE WITH VOMITING, ONE WITH RIGHT LOWER QUADRANT ABDOMINAL PAIN, AND ONE WITH BRIGHT RED RECTAL BLEEDING

Honoria Westphail is a 13 year old girl who was admitted to the hospital because of vomiting, weight loss, and gradually shortening hair braids. The physical examination revealed a slender girl with a somewhat malnourished appearance. There was a mass in the left upper quadrant of the abdomen. A "scout" radiograph of the abdomen (Fig. 83) and an upper G.I. series were performed.

FIGURE 83. Honoria Westphail

FIGURE 84. Grimesby Roylott

Grimesby Roylott, a 15 year old boy from a rural Appalachian area, was referred to the radiology department for an upper G.I. series and small bowel follow-through (Fig. 84) because of cramping, intermittent right lower quadrant abdominal pain. He denied all other symptoms and did not appear ill. The physical examination was normal.

FIGURE 85. Percy Armitage

Percy Armitage is a 13 year old school boy from the eastern shore of Maryland. He was completely well except that one day he noticed bright red blood in the toilet after a bowel movement. His pediatrician could find no cause for the bleeding and referred the child to a radiologist for an air contrast barium enema. (Fig. 85 is a right lateral decubitus radiograph.)

ANSWERS

Honoria Westphail was a somewhat anxious girl with the strange habit of eating her own hair — trichophagia. Figure 83 shows the stomach filled with radiolucent material. After several mouthfuls of barium were swallowed a trichobezoar was outlined by the barium which flowed around it (Fig. 86).

The treatment for a trichobezoar is gastrotomy and removal of the mass. If the trichobezoar extends into the small bowel, it must also be removed to prevent obstruction.

This condition usually occurs in teenage girls who are emotionally disturbed. Honoria has been undergoing psychotherapy while recovering from her surgery. It is expected that this will be continued on an outpatient basis after her discharge from the hospital.

(Rhetorical question: Will trichobezoars become more common in boys with the longer hair styles?)

FIGURE 86.   Honoria Westphail

Grimesby Roylott unknowingly brought a few of his friends with him for a free upper G.I. series. Look closely at the right lower quadrant region and you will see several long cylindrical objects with white streaks running down their middles. These roundworms, *Ascaris lumbricoides*, are making their home in *Grimesby's* small bowel and are ingesting the barium their host has provided. The white streak outlines the gastrointestinal tract of the worm (normal so far as we can tell).

Grimesby was treated with piperazine, the drug of choice for ascariasis. We are not certain that his symptoms were related to the worms, because frequently ascariasis is asymptomatic. At any rate, since treatment *Grimesby* says he feels better.

FIGURE 87.   Grimesby Roylott   Page 70

Percy did not like the preparation for the air contrast barium enema, which consisted of several days of a clear liquid diet, a cathartic, and an enema, but the result was a moderately clean colon in which the polyp and its stalk in the descending colon were clearly identified, free of obscuring feces. Several other shadows were thought to be feces rather than polyps, a distinction difficult to make if the colon is not well prepared.

The radiologist thought that the lesion identified was a juvenile polyp (Fig. 88), although usually such polyps are seen in younger children around the age of 5. Juvenile polyps are not true polyps but are composed largely of fibrous tissue with little overlying epithelium. They are thought to arise from chronic inflammation, perhaps with obstruction of the mucous glands. The juvenile polyp may have a long stalk or a sessile, mushroom-like appearance with a broad base attached to the colonic wall. The force of peristalsis may cause a juvenile polyp to be the lead point of an intussusception. Alternatively, the fecal stream may erode the polyp and cause rectal bleeding.

Juvenile polyps do not resemble the adenomatous polyps of adulthood. They do not become malignant. If left alone, they will slough spontaneously. Surgery is indicated, however, if a juvenile polyp causes excessive bleeding, if it prolapses through the anus, or if it could be shown that the polyp was the lead point of an intussusception.

The most important lesion to exclude in the differential diagnosis of polypoid lesions in children is the adenomatous polyp of familial polyposis. Since one or more of these very numerous polyps will ultimately become malignant, colectomy must be considered. The radiologist and the pediatrician questioned *Percy's* mother about her health and that of her husband, looking for any evidence of a history of familial polyposis or carcinoma of the colon. Because familial polyposis is inherited as a Mendelian dominant trait, and because his parents are normal, it would be relatively unlikely that *Percy* has familial polyposis.

Other conditions that were considered are the Peutz-Jeghers form of intestinal polyposis. This condition is accompanied by melanin spots around the mouth and on the buccal mucosa. These lesions were not found on *Percy*. Gardner's syndrome (multiple polyposis with sebaceous cysts and bony tumors) was dismissed because the last two findings weren't present.

The child was periodically checked to be certain that he did not become anemic due to excessive bleeding. He has had no further bleeding, so the polyp has probably spontaneously sloughed.

FIGURE 88. Percy Armitage

A NEWBORN WITH A BOWEL OBSTRUCTION

FIG. 89

The radiograph in Figure 89 was obtained because of bilious vomiting and abdominal distention in a 24 hour old baby boy named **Watson.** During this time, the baby had not passed any meconium, and it was thought that the baby had an intestinal obstruction at an unknown site. The possibilities included ileal or jejunal atresia, malrotation with volvulus or obstructing bands, Hirschsprung's disease, and meconium ileus.

The supine abdominal radiograph (Fig. 89) showed clearly distended loops of bowel in the left side of the abdomen. In the right lower quadrant of the abdomen, collections of gas are seen interspersed with soft tissue density material, in this case probably meconium (although gas in an abscess might have this appearance). While this is not a finding that is absolutely specific, it is seen when gas in the ileum is forced by peristaltic waves into meconium that is more viscid than normal. The thick, sticky meconium obstructs the ileum and is responsible for the bilious vomiting, abdominal distention, and failure to pass stools.

This condition is known as meconium ileus, and it is only one of the manifestations of cystic fibrosis (also known as mucoviscidosis). This disease is inherited as an autosomal recessive condition which affects the exocrine glands in varying degrees. The mucus secretions are excessively viscid. In the intestines this causes the meconium to become tenacious and leads to a bowel obstruction. In the lungs, the bronchi become obstructed by the thick mucus, and atelectasis and infections occur. In the sinuses, obstructed mucus glands and polyps are found. Obstruction of the bile ducts causes biliary cirrhosis, while the pancreatic ducts are frequently obstructed and the exocrine pancreatic glands gradually degenerate and are replaced by connective tissue.

If the baby has meconium ileus, we can expect the colon to be unused and empty; that is, to have a microcolon appearance.

It has been shown that if water-soluble contrast materials such as Gastrografin or Renografin are used in an enema, the hyperosmolarity of these agents will "pull" water into the gut and may cause the meconium to become more dispersed in the body water–contrast agent mixture with relief of the obstruction.

This diagnostic and therapeutic treatment plan is not used if there are clinical signs of peritonitis, sepsis, or perforation of the intestine or if free air is seen on the preliminary views of the abdomen. It requires recognition that dehydration will occur and that careful control of intravenous fluids is necessary.

ANSWER

When it was clear that *Baby Boy Watson's* condition was stable and additional films made it clear that he had none of the contraindications to contrast study, a Gastrografin enema was given. This showed the small diameter of the bowel characteristic of microcolon (Fig. 90). There was reflux into the terminal ileum, which also had a small caliber and unused appearance. The more proximal gas-filled bowel was dilated, indicating that the bowel obstruction had not been relieved and was either in the jejunum or more proximal ileum. At this point, the baby expelled the Gastrografin and it can be seen outlining the baby's buttocks and back. The child was washed and put in a dry blanket so that he would not get cold and the study repeated several hours later (Fig. 91). At this point, pellets of meconium can be seen in the descending colon. The Gastrografin was refluxed into the ileum and, with continued reflux, finally reached dilated small bowel, which is seen in the right lower quadrant of the abdomen. Soon afterward, *Baby Watson* started to pass meconium. (The baby did not become dehydrated even with the extensive reflux because of the intravenous fluid therapy.)

Had the water-soluble enema not worked, surgery for removal of the meconium would have been necessary. Such surgery has considerable risk and only moderate success. If the bowel is not viable, the necrotic segments are resected.

This form of neonatal bowel obstruction does not have a good prognosis, but as of now *Baby Boy Watson* has been discharged from the hospital in satisfactory condition. The pulmonary complications of cystic fibrosis presumably will develop later in childhood.

FIG. 90

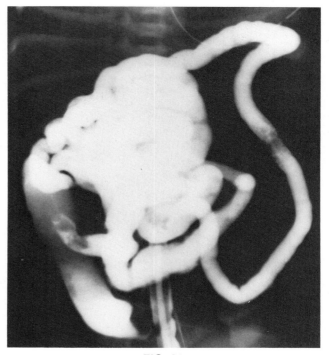

FIG. 91

THE ADVENTURE OF THE DIRTY STOVE

James Moriarty, a 2 year old boy, was seen three weeks ago by his doctor because of coughing, vomiting, and inability to handle secretions for one day.

The doctor examined the boy at that time and diagnosed aphthous stomatitis, or canker sores. He prescribed aspirin and a mouthwash for relief of symptoms.

The day before these radiographs (Figs. 92 and 93) were obtained, *James*
refused to swallow anything, including his saliva. The child was admitted to the hospital, and this barium swallow was performed. It was difficult for the boy to swallow because of pain. The radiologist, one S. Holmes, suggested that Mrs. Moriarty had recently been cleaning her stove, or possibly her sink, toilet, or bathtub. Why?

FIGURE 92. James Moriarty

FIG. 93

ANSWER

Dr. Holmes interpreted the barium swallow as showing the entire length of the esophagus to be diseased. The diameter was narrowed with an irregular contour to the margins. Fluoroscopic examination showed decreased distensibility of the esophagus and normal peristaltic waves which were dampened in amplitude. Dr. Holmes interpreted the changes as indicative of a long esophageal stricture and questioned Mrs. Moriarty about her recent household chores. Apparently, about three weeks before *James* was admitted to the hospital, his mother had been cleaning her stove. There was a small amount of the cleaning agent left in the can when she threw it onto the trash pile in the backyard. A few hours later, the child came running indoors complaining of severe burning in his mouth. The next day he was taken to the doctor and the diagnosis of aphthous stomatitis was made.

The radiographs on the opposite page demonstrate the late changes of a "lye burn" of the esophagus. The cleansing products used for cleaning stoves contain a high percentage of sodium and potassium hydroxide. Usually, burns are seen in the mouth unless the child spits the substance out immediately. No damage is done in the stomach because the alkali is neutralized by hydrochloric acid. In the esophagus lye is in contact with the walls for a long enough time to allow superficial and deep burns to develop. These heal with stricture formation, which is what we see here.

Treatment begins with prevention — keeping such material away from children. After the damage is done, steroid therapy may be used to reduce the inflammation. After strictures have formed, esophageal dilation with bougies is necessary. If that fails, it is sometimes necessary to interpose a segment of the colon between the cervical esophagus and the stomach.

Currently, *James* is undergoing a trial of esophageal dilation with bougies of slowly increasing size. He has continued difficulty with swallowing, and it is thought that he will never have normal pharyngeal and esophageal function.

> It's no doubt clear to everyone by now that the names have been changed to protect the innocent. In this part of the abdominal section, all the names come from the characters in the Sherlock Holmes stories.

FOUR CHILDREN WITH BED-WETTING

Below and on the opposite page are excretory urograms on four children with bed-wetting problems. Their physical examinations are normal, as are their urinalyses. The parents are upset and want the radiologist to find an organic cause for the bed-wetting that can be cured easily and quickly.

FIGURE 94. Charley Once-a-Week

FIGURE 95. Charley Once-a-Week

FIGURE 96. Harry Twice-a-Week

FIGURE 97.   Nancy Nightly

FIGURE 98.   Earl Everyday-but-Sunday

FIGURE 99.   Earl Everyday-but-Sunday

ANSWERS

Charley Once-a-Week's excretory urogram showed two sets of opacified collecting systems on the same side of the spine. No kidney tissue was seen in the right side of the abdomen or in the pelvis. The upper set of calyces appears reasonably normal, but the lower set appears peculiar. Other films showed that the ureters enter the bladder normally.

This is crossed renal ectopia. An ectopic kidney is one that has never reached its normal position. Ectopic kidneys may be fused or nonfused to their mates, and the blood supply may be normal or anomalous. There is an increased incidence of both renal calculi and urinary tract infections in this condition. *Charley Once-a-Week's* parents were disappointed to learn that crossed renal ectopia, by itself, is not the cause of *Charley's* bedwetting. The slight dilatation of the lower pelvis is common and perhaps normal in this condition.

Harry Twice-a-Week's kidneys are fused at their lower poles. The calyces of the right kidney are directed posteriorly and slightly medially, and the right ureter can be seen to be passing laterally. There is probably fusion of renal tissue at the inferior pole of the kidneys, but sometimes only fibrous fusion occurs. The ureters course anteriorly over the fused segment.

Harry has a horseshoe kidney. As in crossed renal ectopia, calculi and infection may be associated with this anomaly. Horseshoe kidney by itself is not a direct cause of bed-wetting, however.

Nancy Nightly, a 6 year old girl, has an entirely normal excretory urogram. The stomach has been distended by giving *Nancy* a carbonated beverage. This distention of the stomach has displaced the small bowel and allowed excellent visualization of the kidneys.

Earl Everyday-but-Sunday has a pelvic kidney, that is, a kidney located within or just above the bony pelvis.

Both *Earl* and *Charley* were first-borns. Their parents were unaware that bladder control could not be expected in a child under the age of 2 years. (Did you notice that *Earl's* and *Charley's* capital femoral epiphyses had not yet appeared? Both children are about 1 year old.)

As for *Nancy* and *Harry*, the cause of their bed-wetting remains unknown. Various organic abnormalities, including spina bifida occulta, and various psychiatric theories have been proposed to explain bed-wetting. Numerous treatments and medications have come into vogue and then faded away. It seems then that usually the cause of bed-wetting is unknown, but certainly there is often a large emotional component of this disorder.

FIVE MORE PATIENTS WITH ABNORMALITIES OF THE URINARY SYSTEM

Baby Boy Geldwasser, 2 days old, had passed only a few drops of urine since birth. The baby did not appear ill, but both kidneys and the bladder were easily palpable. He was referred for a *voiding cystourethrogram*. In performing a "VCUG," a sterile catheter is passed into the bladder and water-soluble contrast material is instilled. As soon as the baby starts to void around the catheter, the catheter is removed and spot films are taken.

Figure 100 demonstrates the narrow caliber of the anterior urethra. The more proximal urethra, the prostatic urethra, is markedly dilated. At the junction of the two segments of urethra are very thin folds of uroepithelium. Usually the folds cannot be seen in the VCUG, but the severe obstruction caused by these posterior urethral valves can be seen. They cause the abrupt change in the caliber of the urethra, so well shown in Figure 100. The valves resemble the cusps of the aortic valve in that upon micturition, they balloon *outward* much as the aortic valve leaflets balloon *inward* during diastole. The posterior urethral valves form an obstruction which leads to bladder distention, diverticulum formation, bilateral ureteral reflux, and bilateral hydronephrosis. Figure 100 demonstrates a bladder diverticulum displacing one ureter posteriorly, and Figure 101 shows the striking hydroureter and left hydronephrosis. Further films showed the hydronephrosis to be bilateral.

Initial treatment consists of relieving the obstruction either by a diversion procedure, such as bilateral nephrostomy or ureterostomy, or by resection of the valves.

FIGURE 100.   Oblique voiding cystourethrogram

FIG. 101

Page 79

FIGURE 102. Stone Henge

Stone Henge, a 6 year old boy, was sent from the Emergency Room to the Radiology Department for an IVP. His mother had brought *Stone* to the hospital because of vomiting, pain in the lower abdomen radiating to the right testicle region, and frequent urination. This was the first such attack.

The physical examination was difficult because the child was in considerable pain and was unable to cooperate. The urinalysis demonstrated WBC's TNTC (too numerous to count) and scattered bacteria.

Pictured here is the preliminary radiograph taken prior to injection of IVP contrast material (Fig. 102).

When **Bobby X.** was born, it was obvious that he had a major abnormality in his genitourinary system. His bladder opened directly onto the lower abdominal wall. The trigone of the bladder as well as both ureteral openings were clearly visible, and the urine spilled out onto the anterior abdominal wall. The penis was foreshortened and epispadias was evident. Figure 103 shows the preliminary view for an IVP.

FIGURE 103. Bobby X.

Phil Hydron, a 6 month old boy, was seen because of a mass in the left upper quadrant of the abdomen. This radiograph (Fig. 104) was obtained five minutes after injection of urographic contrast material. Why is the stomach so distended?

FIGURE 104. Phil Hydron

Ronald Reflux, age 5, has had urinary tract infections much of his life. His x-ray workup has included repeated voiding cystourethrograms and IVP's. Unfortunately, the chart, the radiographs, and the reports are unavailable at the time this IVP is "set up" for interpretation. Should you read the films or put them aside until the previous studies are available? The left kidney appears shrunken, and the calyces are clubbed. Is it enough to simply report the various causes for this radiographic appearance?

FIGURE 105. Ronald Reflux

FIGURE 106. Stone Henge

ANSWERS

Stone's preliminary radiograph suggested that a calculus might be present at the right ureterovesical junction. This is a delayed radiograph (the contrast material has already been propelled out of the left kidney), and it shows distended calyces in the right kidney and opacification of the entire course of the right ureter. The obstruction is incomplete and acute because the excretory function of the right kidney is well preserved. In total acute obstruction there may be little or no detectable urographic function of the affected kidney.

Stone passed the calculus spontaneously. He was treated for his urinary tract infection and evaluated to determine if a cause for the calculus formation could be established. There was no evidence of cystinuria, vitamin D intoxication, hyperparathyroidism, renal tubular acidosis, or sulfonamide therapy. He has not had another urinary tract infection nor has he formed another stone, and the explanation for the formation of this calculus remains unknown.

Bobby X.'s physical findings established the diagnosis of exstrophy of the bladder. Always associated with this anomaly is diastasis of the symphysis pubis (separation and rotation of the pubic bones). The contrast material is spilling out of the bladder onto the abdominal wall. The left kidney is small and has calyces that are crowded together and malformed. These changes were secondary to repeated urinary tract infections.

FIGURE 107. Bobby X.

FIGURE 108. Phil Hydron

Phil's initial radiograph obtained five minutes after contrast material was injected gave insufficient information about the left kidney. A delayed radiograph (seven hours, Fig. 108) shows striking hydronephrosis of the left kidney. This would have been less apparent if the study had been terminated earlier and demonstrates the value of the delayed radiograph in obstructive uropathy.

Why is the stomach distended with gas on the first radiograph? Because the child was fed a carbonated beverage—but we have been through that already.

FIGURE 109. Ronald Reflux

Fortunately, you decided not to read *Ronald's* current IVP until you had previous films for comparison. An earlier IVP (Fig. 109) showed striking dilatation of the calyces of the left kidney. Figure 110 is a "spot film" from a VCUG. (Can you see the catheter in the urethra?) It shows reflux from the bladder into the left ureter.

The role of vesicoureteral reflux in causing renal atrophy and the place of infections in causing reflux (or is it the reflux that allows the infection?) is highly controversial. *Ronald* had both urinary tract infections and vesicoureteral reflux, and his left kidney was small and scarred. In many cases this can be prevented by long-term antibiotic therapy for the infections. Surgery may be needed to reimplant the ureter and prevent further reflux.

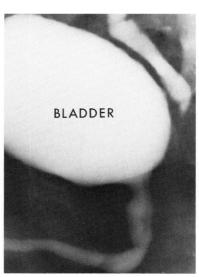

BLADDER

FIGURE 110. Ronald Reflux

A LARGE MASS ON THE BACK OF A NEWBORN

Mrs. Tulp, a 28 year old woman, had been in labor for 22 hours without making progress. The baby began to show signs of fetal distress which necessitated a Caesarean section. The cause for the arrest of labor was found to be a large mass on the back of the baby in the midline, extending from the lower thoracic region to just above the buttocks. Radiographs of the mass, which was protected by a bandage, were obtained as well as skull films. Why were the skull films obtained? What is the diagnosis and what other diagnoses can you establish?

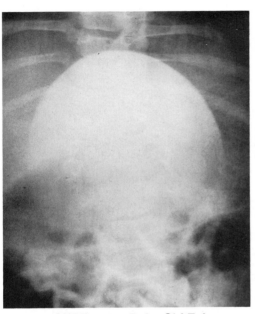

FIGURE 111. Baby Girl Tulp

FIG. 112

FIG. 113

FIG. 114

ANSWERS

Baby Girl Tulp's large mass is well seen in Figure 111 because, being outside the body, it is outlined by air. Look through the mass at the spine. The pedicles are splayed throughout the lumbar region. The extent of the osseous defect is better seen later after the mass had been removed (Fig. 115). The splayed pedicles are seen to extend throughout the lumbar and sacral regions. The change in the appearance of the pedicles is accompanied by widening of the interpediculate distance. *Baby Tulp* has a meningocele; however, if nerve roots or spinal cord are included within the mass, the condition is known as a meningomyelocele.

There was gross neurologic deficit inferior to the mass. The baby dribbled urine occasionally, but no vigorous stream was ever observed. An IVP done when the baby was older (Fig. 116) showed multiple diverticula protruding from an elongated bladder. This is the appearance of a neurogenic bladder.

The radiopaque marker seen over the right acetabulum (Fig. 116) is the tip of a ventriculoperitoneal shunt catheter. A very common finding associated with meningomyelocele is hydrocephalus and Arnold-Chiari malformation. Aqueductal stenosis may also occur with meningocele. These obstructive conditions are treated by diversion procedures such as a ventriculoperitoneal shunt.

The skull radiographs demonstrate thinning of the calvaria; this is especially well seen in the frontal region. The skull has been termed "lacunar skull" or lückenschädel. It is seen almost exclusively in association with meningomyelocele or encephalocele. The local thinning of lacunar skull is much more pronounced than the convolutional marking seen normally.

(Of course you recognize the doughnut-shaped structure seen on the lateral skull radiograph as a roll of adhesive tape!)

FIG. 115

FIG. 116

FIGURE 117. Tom

The following two cases involve children who had excretory urograms performed because of an abdominal mass.

Tom, a 1½ year old boy, had fever, weight loss, and diarrhea lasting four months. Physical examination suggested consolidation in the right lower lobe of the lung. An abdominal film showed a large mass in the right upper quadrant which contained calcifications. An IVP was performed and the relationship of the mass to the kidney suggested the diagnosis. Can you decide what it was?

FIGURE 118. Tom

Ellen, a 7 month old girl, was brought to the hospital because her mother had noticed an abdominal mass while bathing her. She claimed that the mass was not present the previous day. Bleeding into a mass may cause sudden increase in size, making it palpable. After the IVP was studied, a provisional diagnosis and treatment plan was established. How would you interpret the study?

FIGURE 119.   Ellen

FIGURE 120.   Ellen

ANSWERS

Tom's preliminary film shows amorphous calcification in the right upper quadrant of the abdomen. The mass has elevated the right hemidiaphragm. The excretory urogram demonstrates that the internal architecture of the right kidney is normal, but the axis of the kidney has been altered and displaced inferiorly. These findings indicate that the mass is *extrinsic* to the kidney. The calcification seen here is common in neuroblastoma.

Neuroblastomas may arise from the adrenal medulla and also from the sympathetic nervous system. Rarely, a neuroblastoma may change spontaneously to a more benign tumor. Neuroblastomas usually occur before age 4 years, with a maximal incidence at 18 months.

The frequent manifestations of neuroblastoma are abdominal mass, and failure to thrive and gain weight. Many babies will have metastases to the liver or bone at the time of initial examination. The laboratory evaluation includes assessment of urinary degradation products of norepinephrine, dopa, and dopamine. These substances are produced by the neuroblastoma cells and are detectable in the urine in more than nine out of ten cases. Bone marrow biopsy may disclose tumor cells in the marrow cavity long before radiographic changes are apparent.

Treatment is primarily surgical, but radiation therapy and chemotherapy have been shown to markedly increase survival rate. Prognosis is best in patients under the age of 1 year and in those without metastases. Bone involvement which is apparent radiologically indicates a poor prognosis.

Ellen has a large mass in the left upper quadrant of the abdomen. No calcification is present, and no distinguishing features are seen in the mass (except that it indents the stomach air bubble). Urographic contrast material was injected into a foot vein, and AP and lateral views of the abdomen were obtained. No compression, obstruction, or displacement of the inferior vena cava was seen. The following routine IVP radiographs showed that the right kidney appeared normal but that the calyces of the left kidney were markedly distorted and separated.

These findings establish that the mass is an *intrinsic* renal mass. The most common malignant *intrinsic* renal mass of childhood is Wilms' tumor. (Yes, this is spelled correctly — the man's name was Marx Wilms.)

The most common symptom is abdominal mass; however, pain and fever may occur as well as hypertension. The association of Wilms' tumor with hemihypertrophy of both soft tissues and skeleton and aniridia (no iris) is well known, but not commonly seen.

The workup may be supplemented with angiography to demonstrate the extent of the tumor and to determine if there is growth of the neoplasm into the renal vein and inferior vena cava. If this is found, measures can be taken to prevent tumor emboli from reaching the lungs. In this regard, if Wilms' tumor is suspected clinically, palpation of the abdomen should be kept to a minimum.

Treatment of Wilms' tumor is aimed at primary excision of the tumor with the capsule intact. Post-operative radiotherapy has been found to increase the number of survivors. Chemotherapy, notably actinomycin D, also increases the survival rate, and both chemotherapy and radiotherapy are used in most treatment plans currently. When metastases occur in Wilms' tumor, the lungs and liver are common sites, but the bones are rarely involved.

It should be added that the use of ultrasound in the differentiation of abdominal masses is becoming increasingly important.

. . . NOW YOU OUGHT TO BE READY
TO INTERPRET THIS EXCRETORY UROGRAM:

FIGURE 121. Sam Trail, 5 years old

FIGURE 122. Sam T.

Sam T. was 5 years old when all radiographs shown here were obtained. AP and lateral skull films (Figs. 122 and 123) demonstrated marked diastasis of the coronal and sagittal sutures and bone destruction. These changes are caused by metastatic neuroblastoma to the dura and cranium.

The chest radiograph (Fig. 124) demonstrates lytic changes in virtually all the bones. At the same time, notice that no metastatic deposits are visible in the lungs—pulmonary metastases are uncommon with neuroblastoma.

FIGURE 123. Sam T.

FIGURE 124. Sam T.

The radiographs of the arms (Fig. 125) show the symmetrical character of the metastases. Symmetrical metastatic deposits are one of the hallmarks of this condition.

The IVP (Fig. 121) shows displacement of the right kidney from its normal axis by a mass superior to it. The calcification in the right upper quadrant was a key finding (Fig. 126, detail); together with the bone changes in the pelvis, this one film establishes that the mass is most likely a **neuroblastoma.**

FIGURE 125. Sam T., right and left arms

FIGURE 126. Sam T.

SKULL

SEIZURES DIFFICULT TO CONTROL AND MENTAL RETARDATION

FIGURE 127.   Mary Beth

Mary Beth (Fig. 127), age 7, had been referred to the Seizure Clinic because of increasing frequency of seizures. Her condition was recognized at birth on the basis of a purple cutaneous lesion (port-wine hemangioma) that was distributed over the area innervated by the right trigeminal nerve. *Mary Beth* was 1 year old when left-sided grand mal seizures began. Recently the seizures have occurred more frequently.

The neurologic examination demonstrated a spastic left hemiparesis and a visual field deficit. Skull radiographs confirmed the diagnosis (Figs. 128, 129, and 130).

FIGURE 129. Towne's projection: Mary Beth

FIGURE 128. Frontal projection: Mary Beth

FIGURE 130. Lateral projection: Mary Beth

ANSWER

Mary Beth's skull radiographs demonstrate railroad track calcification extending from the occipital pole to the frontal pole of the right cerebral cortex. This is calcification of the shrunken cerebral cortical gyri. These are *not* the calcified walls of blood vessels. The port-wine hemangioma seen on the face has its counterpart in venous angiomatosis of the pia and arachnoid layers of the meninges overlying the affected area.

This is *encephalofacial angiomatosis*, or the Sturge-Weber syndrome. The affected portion of the cerebral hemisphere may be significantly smaller than its mate, resulting in failure of growth of the overlying calvaria and an asymmetrical skull.

Visual field deficit, hemiparesis, seizures, and mental retardation are clinical manifestations of the cerebral atrophy and dysfunction. Treatment is aimed at reducing the frequency of seizures with anticonvulsant medication. If the seizures aren't controlled medically, surgical excision of the affected cortex may be considered.

FIGURE 131.   Another case of Sturge-Weber syndrome with less extensive calcification of the cerebral cortex

ANOTHER PROBLEM: MULTIPLE WORMIAN BONES

Notice the multiple bones in the lambdoidal suture in the patient illustrated in Figure 132, **Frank Fragile.** These bones are known as wormian bones (after the Danish anatomist Olaus Worm—not after helminths). They are areas of ossification of membranous bone which arise in the sutures and fontanelles. When there are multiple wormian bones, several conditions should come to mind. What are they?

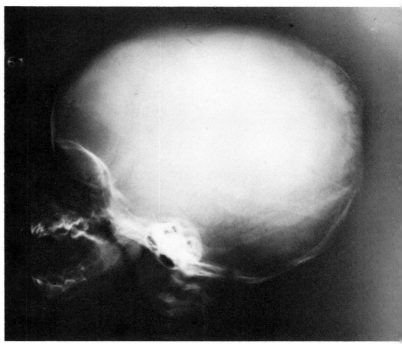

FIG. 132

ANSWER

Frank Fragile, a 1 year old boy, was dropped from a table, striking his head on the floor. Figures 132 and 133 show radiographs taken before and after the trauma. The first shows the wormian bones, but something has been added on the second study—multiple lucent lines. These are **skull fractures.** *Frank Fragile* has blue sclera, multiple wormian bones, and many skull and skeletal fractures. He has **osteogenesis imperfecta.**

Other conditions with multiple wormian bones include cretinism, cleidocranial dysostosis, and hypophosphatasia.

FIG. 133

INTRACRANIAL CALCIFICATION

FIGURE 134. Paul C.

One of the common reasons pediatricians obtain skull radiographs of infants is to aid in the evaluation of slow development. **Paul C.**, a 4 year old boy, had not yet begun to talk or walk. His head was large for his body and his forehead was especially prominent.

The radiographs suggest the cause of failure of normal growth and development. What special procedures would you use to prove the *diagnosis*? (The oblique lines projected over the left orbit and across the top of the skull are artifacts. What are they?)

FIGURE 135. Paul C.

Harvey B., a 28 month old boy, was sent by his ophthalmologist for skull radiographs because of the finding of chorioretinitis. What finding did the ophthalmologist think the radiographs might demonstrate?

FIGURE 136. Harvey B.

FIGURE 137. Harvey B.

FIGURE 138.   Paul C.

FIGURE 139.   Paul C.

ANSWERS

Paul C.'s skull radiographs demonstrate calcification that appears symmetrical and conforms to the expected margins of dilated lateral ventricles. The next step to test this hypothesis might be a pneumoencephalogram (Figs. 138 and 139). These radiographs confirm the location of the calcification in the walls of dilated lateral ventricles. The excessively wide sulci are outlined by air and indicate brain atrophy. *Paul* has cytomegalic inclusion disease, a viral illness that may be acquired during gestation. Congenital CID infection may affect the lungs, liver, and hematopoietic system as well as the central nervous system. Unfortunately, there is no treatment for this disease.

The lines projected across *Paul's* forehead and left orbit are pieces of adhesive tape used to immobilize the patient. (An edge is seen when there is an air–adhesive tape interface.)

Harvey B.'s skull radiographs show calcification distributed throughout the brain. This type and distribution of calcification is seen in another congenital infection, toxoplasmosis. Toxoplasma is a parasite which can sometimes be demonstrated in the cerebrospinal fluid. If the baby is not stillborn, he may be left with brain damage, microcephaly, seizures, and chorioretinitis. In this patient, the basis for the chorioretinitis was indeed toxoplasmosis.

The periventricular distribution of calcification seen in *Paul* and the diffuse distribution seen with *Harvey* are not absolutely specific for the etiologic agent. However the calcification does indicate a congenital infection and suggests the *likely* pathogen.

SUPRASELLAR CALCIFICATION

Karen L., a 3 year old girl, was seen initially by her pediatrician because of persistent vomiting and headache. Physical examination demonstrated papilledema, and *Karen* was admitted to the hospital where skull radiographs were obtained. The lateral radiograph (Fig. 140) shows calcification above the sella turcica. The sella itself is enlarged with undermining of the anterior clinoid processes and thinning of the dorsum. The coronal sutures are diastatic. What is the diagnosis?

ANSWER

Karen has a craniopharyngioma. This is a histologically benign cystic tumor which arises from epithelium that contributes to the formation of the pituitary gland. The squamous cell component of the hypophysis is slowly shed and accumulates to form a cystic mass. The expansion of this mass interrupts the flow of CSF toward the cerebral convexities, causing hydrocephalus, increased intracranial pressure, papilledema, headache, vomiting, and widened sutures. Calcification occurs in the necrotic debris of shed cells and is almost always present in children with craniopharyngioma. Visual field defects occur because of direct pressure on the optic pathways.

The aim of therapy is total excision of the craniopharyngioma. The size and location of the tumor may make this quite difficult. Furthermore, interruption of pituitary function is expected (reduced ACTH formation, diabetes insipidus, etc.). It may not be possible to remove the entire craniopharyngioma, and it is sometimes necessary to reoperate when the symptoms return.

FIG. 140

SEIZURES AND MENTAL RETARDATION
BE CAREFUL: ALL THAT GLITTERS IS NOT GOLD (OR CALCIUM)

FIGURE 141. Bobby Bogus

Bobby Bogus, 3 years old, was clearly retarded. He also had seizures and was admitted for manipulation of anticonvulsive drug dosage as well as for determination of the basis for the seizures and mental retardation. Included here are AP and lateral skull radiographs. What procedure did *Bobby* have just before the skull radiographs were taken?

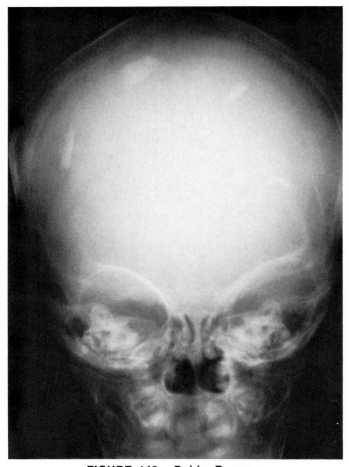

FIGURE 142. Bobby Bogus

F. Fake, age 2, has the same history as *Bobby Bogus. F.* in this case is a female name *(Frieda)*. How can we be certain? What are the serpentine shadows projected over the parietal region on the lateral skull radiographs (Fig. 143)?

FIGURE 143. F. Fake

ANSWERS

At first glance *Bobby Bogus* seems to have multiple areas of intracranial calcification. It's somewhat difficult to think of a disease that causes this pattern of calcification. In fact, *Bobby* had an electroencephalogram just prior to coming to the Pediatric Radiology department for his skull series. The densities seen projected over the calvaria are caused by EEG paste, which is used to insure good conductivity between the scalp and the "EEG leads." The proof is in the shampoo. After *Bobby* was shampooed the "calci-

fications" disappeared. (*Bobby's* final diagnosis was idiopathic epilepsy, which has no roentgen findings.)

We can tell *Frieda Fake* is a female because of the serpentine shadows seen on the lateral skull radiographs. These are tightly wound hair braids, a style very popular with black girls.

Artifacts ("made by hand") are a very real part of radiology. It's not enough to recognize the abnormal. You must be able to separate what simulates the abnormal from what is genuinely pathologic.

TWO PATIENTS WITH UNUSUAL HEAD SHAPE

FIG. 144

At age 3 months, **Sheila T.** was noticed to have an asymmetrical face with a flattened left side of the forehead and orbit region. In retrospect, the parents thought that this deformity had been present since birth.

The child appeared otherwise well, and the neurologic examination was negative. These skull radiographs were obtained (Figs. 144 and 145).

FIG. 145

FIG. 146

Harold W., age 5, was seen by a pediatric neurologist because of hyperactive behavior and the question of minimal brain damage. He had been born with a long, egg-shaped skull, but no one had thought this remarkable. These skull radiographs were obtained as part of the neurologic workup (Figs. 146, 147, and 148).

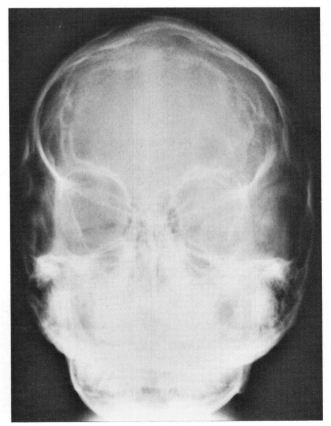

FIG. 148

FIG. 147

ANSWERS

Sheila T.'s orbits are asymmetrical. The right orbit is round, whereas the left orbital rim is triangular; the orbital roof is elevated and points upward and outward. The lateral view is obliqued enough so that the coronal suture region on each side of the skull can be separately evaluated. No portion of the coronal suture is visible.

Sheila has premature synostosis of at least the left half of the coronal suture (judging from the orbital deformity). Because the lateral radiograph failed to demonstrate either limb of the coronal suture well, the surgeons elected to perform a bilateral excision of a strip of the calvaria in the region of the coronal sutures. To retard regrowth of bone, a polyethylene film was folded over the bone at the edges of the defect and left in place (Fig. 149).

The generic term for premature closure of the sutures is **cranio-synostosis.** Normally, the newborn baby will have the cranial bones separated from each other by the sutures, which at first are merely broad strips of unossified membrane. If two or more of the calvarial bones fuse together, obliterating the suture(s), before birth or during the first few years of life, normal brain growth unduly widens those sutures that are still patent, leading to calvarial deformity. The descriptive terminology is confusing for those untutored in Greek. However, the following chart lists the important and frequently used terms for the cranial malformations due to craniosynostosis. Since the English terms describe the central pathogenetic state (whereas the Greek terms merely refer to the resulting shape, which anyone can figure out), column one probably should be used preferentially.

English	*Greek*	*Meaning*
Unilateral coronal synostosis	Plagiocephaly	Asymmetrical or twisted head
Bilateral coronal synostosis	Brachycephaly	Short head
Sagittal synostosis	Scaphocephaly	Skiff(boat)-shaped long, narrow head
Premature fusion of the sagittal and the coronal *or* occasionally the lambdoid sutures	Oxycephaly	Pointed head

FIGURE 149. Sheila T.

Harold W. has a markedly elongated skull with obliteration of the normal sagittal suture. The bony fusion is well seen on the coned-down (sagittal) detail view in Figure 148. This is sagittal synostosis, or scaphocephaly, and this is the most common suture involved in craniosynostosis.

The indication for surgery in *Harold's* case was cosmetic repair of his odd skull shape, although at his age, alteration in head shape probably will be minimal. More importantly, if several sutures are involved, surgery is generally thought to be indicated for relief of restriction of brain growth which, if untreated, would result in compression, gross distortion of the brain, probable neurologic deficit, and mental retardation. Although the extent of neurologic deficit is thought to be a function of the number of sutures involved, we have seen many children who are mentally normal despite skulls seriously deformed from premature fusion of all calvarial sutures. Possibly, brain and neurologic abnormalities in children with craniosynostosis represent associated malformations and are not the result of craniosynostosis. In *Harold's* case, sagittal synostosis alone would be unlikely to produce any neurologic impairment or mental retardation. In general, however, the greater the number of sutures that are closed, the higher the incidence of mental retardation and neurologic deficit.

Harold had a strip of bone removed from either side of the midline from just anterior to the coronal suture to just behind the lambdoidal suture (Figs. 150 and 151). A midline strip of bone was not removed because bleeding could be a problem if the sagittal sinus were inadvertently lacerated.

In *Harold's* case, the cosmetic results were not as striking as

FIGURE 150.   Harold W.

FIGURE 151.   Harold W.

might have been expected had he been operated upon during the first year of life.

Sheila T. on the other hand appears somewhat improved clinically, whereas untreated, her condition would have worsened.

HOLES IN THE HEAD

FIGURE 152. Hans, age 2

Hans S. was 2 years old when this set of skull radiographs was obtained (Figs. 152 and 153). He was irritable and seemed to have pain on palpation of his head. This was not unexpected because approximately 1 year earlier when the boy had a chronically draining left ear accompanied by a skin eruption that resembled seborrheic dermatitis, radiographs of the skull and of the mastoid region were obtained (Fig. 154).

The diagnosis was made by biopsy of one of the skull lesions, and treatment was initiated. At age 3, however, *Hans* developed loose deciduous molars in the left side of the mandible. Radiographs shown in Figures 155 and 156 were obtained. (Fig. 155 is the right side of the mandible and is the normal control.)

What is the diagnosis?

FIGURE 153. Hans, age 2

FIGURE 154.   Hans, age 1

This is the Towne's view of the skull. The hole in the center is the foramen magnum. Seen through it is the incompletely fused arch of the first cervical vertebra. On either side of the foramen magnum are the petrous pyramids. Are they both abnormal?

These oblique views (Figs. 155 and 156) of the mandible have been obtained so that each side of the mandible can be studied separately. A true lateral view of the mandible would superimpose the right and left sides and the overlap would make interpretation difficult.

FIGURE 155.   Hans, age 3

FIGURE 156.   Hans, age 3

ANSWER

Hans S. was originally evaluated because of what was thought to be seborrheic dermatitis and left otitis media. This is not an uncommon manner of presentation for this condition.

The skull radiographs at that time showed a single punched out lesion of bone with a smooth border. This was biopsied, and the specimen showed histiocytes, reticulum cells, and eosinophils. This was thought to represent histiocytosis X.

The Towne's view shows extensive destruction of the left mastoid. Treatment consisted of radiation therapy to the involved area and then chemotherapy. However, at age 3, *Hans* complained of loose teeth in the left side of the mandible. The radiograph (Fig. 156) of the affected area demonstrates the "floating teeth sign," which occurs when there is extensive bone destruction and the teeth are no longer firmly rooted.

Hans has extensive osseous involvement of the skull as well as involvement of the viscera. There is no evidence of pulmonary involvement yet, but *Hans* has anemia, lymph node enlargement, and hepatosplenomegaly. The lytic lesions in the skull (Figs. 152 and 153) are obvious, but did you notice the destruction of the posterior wall of the left orbit? Exophthalmos is beginning to develop.

Histiocytosis X is the generic name for three conditions previously thought to be distinct diseases. Now many authorities consider them to represent different manifestations of the same disease.

Eosinophilic granuloma has the best prognosis of these three diseases. It usually is a disease restricted to one or a few bones. Hand-Schüller-Christian disease may be manifested by (1) unilateral exophthalmos, (2) diabetes insipidus and, (3) skeletal lesions. This triad appears more commonly on examinations than it does clinically and is worth memorizing *only* for that reason. But this is what Hans has.

The least favorable outcome occurs in the Letterer-Siwe condition. This phase of histiocytosis X may be rapidly fatal. Its hallmark is visceral involvement as well as skeletal lesions. The pulmonary changes are not specific by themselves but may resemble pulmonary fibrosis or focal infiltrates. (It may be helpful to study very carefully the corners of the chest radiograph in such a patient for clues such as hepatosplenomegaly or bone destruction and to examine the axilla and cervical regions for enlarged lymph nodes.)

Another manifestation of histiocytosis X not illustrated here is vertebra plana. If you see a patient with a wafer thin vertebra, think of histiocytosis X.

EITHER YOU RECOGNIZE THIS CONDITION AT A GLANCE OR YOU HAVE NO IDEA WHAT IT IS

This case is an example of "pattern recognition," and once you've seen an example, you won't forget it.

Leo de O., age 9, was seen because of an asymmetrical face, and these radiographs were obtained. What's the diagnosis?

ANSWER

The radiographs show a dense area of sclerosis involving the left sphenoid wing and maxillary bone. Bony encroachment has deformed the left maxillary sinus. No skin lesions were seen, and no other abnormalities of bone were identified on a skeletal survey.

This is **monostotic fibrous dysplasia.** In adults, it may be confused with the sclerotic phase of Paget's disease, blastic metastatic deposits, or rarely a very extensive meningioma. In childhood, craniofacial monostotic fibrous dysplasia is distinctive. It usually ceases activity at puberty, does not become malignant, and does not become transformed into polyostotic fibrous dysplasia or Albright's syndrome. In Albright's syndrome the bone changes of fibrous dysplasia are accompanied by café au lait spots and precocious puberty in females. This condition is distinct from *Leo de O.'s* monostotic fibrous dysplasia (but may perhaps be related metabolically).

FIGURE 157. Leo de O.

FIGURE 158. Leo de O.

VOMITING AND HEADACHE

FIGURE 159. Stephen D.

FIGURE 160. Stephen D.

Here is a 10 year old boy, **Stephen D.,** with truly disabling headaches accompanied by vomiting.

The pediatrician found bilateral papilledema and obtained skull radiographs (Figs. 159 and 160). These views are alarming because the sutures are obviously wide (diastatic). The lucent regions in the calvaria are not as useful a sign of increased intracranial pressure as the wide sutures because only slightly less marked lucencies are occasionally seen in the normal child. Note also that the dorsum is thinned and demineralized. This is a reliable sign of increased intracranial pressure, but in children below the age of 8 to 12 the still-open sutures are a more sensitive index of changes in intracranial pressure and will become abnormal before the sella does.

The problem, then, resolves itself into organization of a differential diagnosis of increased intracranial pressure in a 10 year old. We use the acronym TINC to help remember some of the causes of increased intracranial pressure.

The T stands for *trauma*. A child may have suffered trauma sufficiently severe to cause bilateral subdural hematomas without producing a skull fracture.

I is for *infection*, notably brain abscess, seen commonly in children with cyanotic congenital heart disease and in children with meningitis of any cause.

N is the first letter of *neoplasm*. Under this heading are included cerebellar medulloblastoma, brain stem and higher level gliomas, craniopharyngiomas, and papilloma of the choroid plexus.

The C of *congenital* is the last heading. Included in this group are aqueductal stenosis, Arnold-Chiari malformation (think of this if there is a meningomyelocele), and Dandy-Walker syndrome (atresia of the foramina of Luschka and Magendie, causing great enlargement of the fourth and higher ventricles).

Actually this scheme is not complete. For example, in what category would you place thrombosis of the sagittal sinus, or "pseudo-tumor cerebri" (benign increased intracranial pressure)?

ANSWER

Stephen D. had a complete workup including thorough history and physical examination as well as lumbar puncture, complete blood count, blood culture, brain scan, EEG, and a ventriculogram, which demonstrated aqueductal stenosis. The head size is within normal limits; however, the sutures are quite wide, indicating that the increased pressure is of recent onset. *Stephen* thus did not have typical congenital aqueductal stenosis with evidence of increased intracranial pressure starting at or before birth. Possibly, his was acquired and secondary to hemorrhage or infection, although this is uncertain.

A ventriculoperitoneal shunt was performed (Fig. 161). Notice that there is a radiopaque tubing with a dense marker at its tip.

This is connected to a valve-flushing device combination that looks like a button in this illustration. The tubing is then tunneled through the superficial layers of the neck and chest into the peritoneal cavity where the CSF is drained and reabsorbed.

The shunting procedure has resulted in diminished intracranial pressure, and the sutures and sella turcica appear normal. As the intracranial pressure decreases, sometimes a collection of blood develops in the epidural space. Normally, the intracranial pressure will tamponade such an accumulation, but the shunt device transmits the pressure to the peritoneal cavity and the epidural collection can expand. The calcified biconvex density seen in the posterior parietal region (Fig. 161 and detail in Fig. 162) is a calcified epidural hematoma. (The densities projected over the sella turcica are particles of Pantopaque, a contrast agent used in the earlier ventriculogram.)

FIGURE 161.   Stephen D.

FIGURE 162.   Stephen D.

MASS ON FOREHEAD

FIGURE 163. Baby Thomas

Baby Thomas was obviously malformed at birth inasmuch as a huge soft tissue mass protruded anteriorly from the midline of the forehead. This mass was so large that the eyes were separated (hypertelorism), creating a most unusual appearance. This mass was found not to transilluminate with light. On the opposite page are two special procedures done prior to surgery.

What is your preoperative diagnosis?

ANSWER

The preoperative diagnosis was anterior encephalocele. One of the considerations helpful to the surgeons is the determination of the contents of the mass. Is there simply a small amount of dysplastic brain surrounded by fluid, or is the amount of brain much more substantial?

The ventriculogram (Fig. 164) demonstrates extension of a lateral ventricle into the mass. The amount of cerebral tissue seems substantial. The angiogram demonstrates the blood supply and also helps determine the amount of brain substance included in the encephalocele.

Surgery was performed utilizing an intracranial approach in the excision of the herniated and malformed brain. A tantalum plate covered the osseous defect. Later a diversionary procedure was necessary because of hydrocephalus (Fig. 166). *Baby Thomas* has done well since surgery, and seems to have only moderate mental retardation.

Meningomyelocele is much more common than encephalocele. Among encephaloceles, furthermore, the anterior encephaloceles are much less common than occipital encephaloceles. If an occipital encephalocele is present, not only cerebellum but also cerebral tissue may be herniated into the sac. A frontal encephalocele may protrude into the nose, simulating a nasal polyp, or may extend through the orbit, causing unilateral exophthalmos.

Surgery is indicated not only to prevent infection but also for removal of the unsightly mass.

FIG. 164

FIG. 165

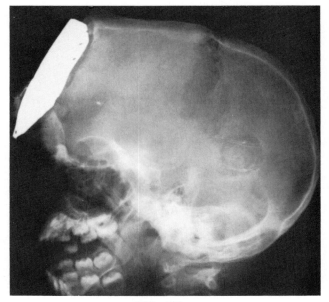

FIG. 166

TWO INFANTS WITH HEAD TRAUMA

FIGURE 167. Tyrone F.

Tyrone F., age 4 months, was brought to the Emergency Room by his nearly hysterical mother. The history was obtained between self-recriminations and sobs, and it seems that while *Tyrone* was having his diaper changed, he fell from the table onto the floor, striking his head.

Physical examination at the time of initial evaluation in the Emergency Room demonstrated that the child appeared well except for moderate soft tissue swelling in the right posterior parietal region. The pupils were of equal size and both reacted to light. The remainder of the neurologic examination and the state of consciousness were normal. A set of skull radiographs was obtained and included Figures 167 and 168.

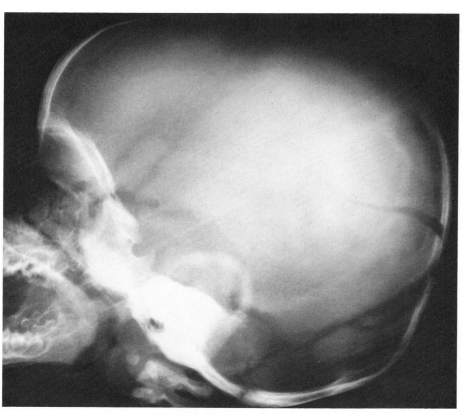

FIGURE 168. Tyrone F.

Patsy D., age 8 months, was also brought to the Emergency Room by her mother, who seemed quite calm and almost apathetic. She said the baby had been somewhat lethargic and had lost her appetite for the past week. She thought that the infant "might have hit her head" against the side of her crib a few days ago.

Physical examination showed an irritable infant who preferred to be left alone. There were ecchymoses over the head, legs, and buttocks. The pupils were equal in size and reacted to light, but the fundi could not be adequately examined because the child was too irritable. (The pediatrician did not use mydriatrics to dilate the pupils, becaust he would then have lost the ability to use inequality of pupils as a reliable sign of intracranial trauma.)

The sutures felt somewhat diastatic and the anterior fontanelle was bulging. No skull fracture (or depressed skull fracture in particular) could be palpated. The skull radiographs were obtained because the history and physical examination raised the suspicion of *significant intracranial trauma.*

FIGURE 169. Patsy D.

FIGURE 170. Patsy D.

ANSWERS

Tyrone F. has a skull fracture in the right posterior parietal region. No depression of the skull fracture fragments is seen, and the sutures appear normal.

Tyrone, in fact, appeared in no great distress. His state of consciousness was normal, as were his vital signs. He was not admitted to the hospital and his parents were instructed to awaken him every two hours throughout the night to determine if he was asleep, or if he had possibly lapsed into coma. They were also instructed how to evaluate pupil size and were told to bring the child back to the Emergency Room immediately if they detected any inequality in pupil diameter. However, *Tyrone* developed no signs of brain injury and has recovered completely.

Patsy D.'s radiographs (Figs. 169 and 170) show no skull fracture. Instead, there is a more ominous finding —diastasis of the sutures. Figure 170 is a Towne's view. The coronal suture, seen just superior to the foramen magnum on this radiograph, is greatly widened. The anterior fontanelle is superimposed on the middle of the occipital bone. The thin lucent lines radiating laterally from the foramen magnum are the synchondroses between the supra-occipital and exoccipital portions of the occipital bone. These are normal findings at this age.

Because of the presence of ecchymoses on other areas of the body, a skeletal survey was made to discover any evidence of trauma in the form of recent or healed fractures. No fractures were seen, but the history of hitting the head against the crib didn't seem compatible with a severe enough injury to produce diastatic sutures; therefore, the battered child syndrome (or "trauma X syndrome") was considered. In addition, the bulging fontanelle and the diastatic sutures indicated that bilateral subdural taps might be helpful. These procedures were performed, and bilateral subdural hematomas were found. Throughout the course of the next several days the child had repeated subdural taps and more fluid was removed.

In retrospect, it seems likely that there had been definite head trauma during which the skull stopped moving immediately and the brain and dural attachments decelerated less rapidly. It is not surprising, then, that some of the vessels were torn, causing a collection of subdural blood, diastasis of the sutures, and bulging of the anterior fontanelle.

The day following *Patsy's* admission to the hospital, it was learned that a sibling had just been found dead at home after "falling down" a flight of stairs. The autopsy showed more than 60 ecchymoses on the child as well as liver and spleen lacerations. The evidence for battered child syndrome (see page 121) was overwhelming, and *Patsy* was not sent home but was discharged to a chronic care facility.

The question of when radiographs of the skull are indicated in head trauma is clouded by the spurious concept of "medicolegal indications." It is argued by some that if a skull series is not obtained and later something is found, a malpractice suit may result. This argument is even extrapolated to such a point that a skull series is obtained on all children with head trauma, whether mild, moderate, or severe. The result is that a tremendous number of children are radiographed with little expectation of yielding any important findings. The cost to parents and welfare agencies is astronomical, especially in proportion to the yield. A more economic approach, which reduces radiation exposure to the child, is the common sense approach: *If the sutures are palpably widened, if a depressed fracture is felt, if the child has evidence of severe head trauma or is unconscious, then radiographs are indicated, but for medical reasons, not legal reasons.* To allow legal considerations to dictate medical practice is unhealthy for the patient in terms of needless radiation exposure and is unnecessarily costly for society.

BONE

TENDER SWELLING IN THE LEFT THIGH

Jill M., age 3 months, was brought to the emergency room by her mother who stated, "My baby has a swollen leg." She could not think what might have caused this, although she recalled that *Jill* seemed to have "twisted her leg in the crib" several days previously.

Physical examination showed a thin, almost emaciated baby obviously in pain. She held her left leg in flexion, and resisted any attempt to move it. The swelling was confirmed, and radiographs of both extremities were obtained (Figs. 171 and 172).

ANSWER

The view of the left thigh shows a hard-to-see slender black line crossing the femur obliquely between the middle and lower thirds (compare to the child's normal right femur). This is a spiral fracture with no separation—a *recent* fracture since no callus is seen.

The comparison view of the right leg reveals a surprising finding. There is a fracture of the right tibia surrounded by abundant callus: hence, this is an *old* fracture. Notice also the irregularity of the most distal end of the tibia. This metaphyseal fraying is due to avulsion of the insertion of the periosteum.

A skeletal survey was obtained and showed anterior compression of the fourth lumbar vertebra, and to a lesser degree, of the third lumbar vertebra (Fig. 173). The baby was admitted to the hospital with a diagnosis of *battered child syndrome,* i.e., child abuse.

FIGURE 171. Jill M.

FIGURE 172. Jill M.

As radiologists we think of this diagnosis if we see the metaphyseal avulsions demonstrated in *Jill's* right tibia. If we have evidence for *fractures of different ages*, the battered child syndrome is almost certainly the explanation.

"Who did it?" is always a problem. This syndrome has been studied in great detail. Batterers come from all levels of society. Only a small number are clearly psychotic. The vast majority of child abusers are not profoundly mentally ill, but one common thread that unites them is their exasperation and frustration with their children.

The battering takes place commonly when the baby is most frustrating: when he cries continuously and nothing will quiet him. At this point the baby is least satisfying, and he is rebuked for being "bad" by being physically abused.

The pediatrician recognizes the battered child by evidence of ecchymoses on the skin, contusions of the gums where a feeding bottle has been jammed into the mouth, hemorrhages into the retina secondary to cranial trauma, and so forth. A more subtle problem is to recognize the battered child with a less obvious manner of presentation, such as "failure to thrive" without obvious cause. Frequently, these children will thrive and gain weight when hospitalized, whereas the normal child usually does just the reverse.

Treatment should therefore begin with hospitalization. The parents are not confronted with the term "child-batterer"; this would be counter-productive. Instead, therapy consists of trying to help the parents cope with their frustrations. Sometimes it is not safe to allow the child to return home, and a foster home must be sought, via the courts if necessary. Other times, gradual return of the child to the home environment can be achieved.

Jill's case was somewhat unusual, since the mother was mentally ill and *Jill* was initially sent to a chronic care facility while her mother received treatment. Only recently has the child returned home for three days a week. The remainder of the time she lives with a close relative. She is followed quite closely by a group caring for children with the battered child syndrome, and there has been no evidence of recurrence.

FIGURE 173.   Jill M.

MORE PEDIATRIC TRAUMA . . .

Paula B., age 7, fell onto her right hand while skipping rope. AP and lateral radiographs of the wrist were obtained (Figs. 174 and 175).

ANSWER

Paula has a fracture of the distal end of the radius and ulna and anterior tilting of the distal fracture fragments. This suggests that her hand was held in volar flexion and was bent forward when she fell. (A boy will fall usually with his hand held in dorsal extension causing the fracture fragments to be displaced dorsally.)

The fracture lines are not well seen because the fractures are impacted. However, the cortical buckling and deformity of alignment indicates that a fracture of the radius and ulna have occurred.

This type of fracture is common and may be quite subtle. It is important to scrutinize the cortex of the distal radius and ulna for a minimal buckle before telling the parents that their child doesn't have a fracture.

FIG. 174

FIG. 175

AND MORE . . .

Henry S., age 8 months, has been crawling all over his play pen with great vigor and has begun to use his legs more and more in an attempt to stand. Today, however, he stopped moving his left leg entirely, and an area of tenderness and erythema was noted. Radiographs of the region were obtained (Figs. 176 and 177).

ANSWER

Henry has a "toddler's fracture," a spiral or oblique fracture of the distal left tibia. This type of injury may occur as the child is learning to walk. It frequently presents as a sudden and adamant refusal to walk or bear weight in an otherwise healthy child; the injury itself may have been unobserved. Sometimes the fractures are so fine that they cannot be seen on the initial radiographs but are visible on films made one to two weeks after the injury, when slight resorption of bone has occurred at the fracture margins, and the periosteum has begun to lay down new bone. In Henry's case, it was not associated with any evidence of the battered child syndrome.

FIG. 176   **FIG. 177**

Henry S.

A CONDITION THAT RADIOLOGICALLY RESEMBLES THE BATTERED CHILD SYNDROME

Pauline F., a 2 month old white female, was admitted to the hospital from the outpatient clinic because of swelling of the left wrist. She had been a 1700-gram premature baby, the product of a pregnancy that was complicated by a red, splotchy cutaneous eruption in the mother during the third trimester. This was not investigated or treated.

The delivery was normal, and the baby remained in the hospital for three weeks, gaining weight. The baby did well at home until now.

Examination in the outpatient clinic showed *Pauline* to be a very small baby who held her left arm limp and cried continuously. Her liver and spleen were large. A lumbar puncture, CBC, urinalysis, and skeletal survey (Figs. 178, 179, and 180) were performed. A bone marrow aspirate clinched the diagnosis, although the radiographs were virtually specific for this condition, which is . . . ?

FIG. 178

FIG. 179

FIG. 180

ANSWER

The outstanding features of the radiographs are the spectacular periosteal reaction in multiple bones, the metaphyseal destruction, and the pathologic fractures. This is not the fine bilaterally symmetrical periosteal elevation that is sometimes seen in the normal newborn and young infant. Instead, this is a gross asymmetrical periosteal cloaking accompanied by metaphyseal destruction never seen in the benign periosteal reaction in the newborn.

As you suspected, *Pauline* has *congenital syphilis*. Sometimes, in this condition along the medial aspect of the proximal ends of the tibias there may be symmetrical areas of destruction which are known as Wimberger's sign of congenital syphilis. The left tibia shows changes that resemble "Wimberger's sign," but usually the metaphyseal destruction is more flagrant. The bone changes of congenital syphilis may also be seen in the calvarium, and the small bones of the hands and feet.

Because the diagnosis of congenital syphilis was radiologically extremely likely, the serologic test for syphilis was performed on the parents and the baby. Both the mother and *Pauline* had markedly positive titers — but these were not immediately available.

The bone marrow aspiration mentioned earlier revealed spirochetes characteristic of treponemes. This procedure is not one of the usual diagnostic tests in the evaluation of a patient with congenital syphilis; it was done here to exclude congenital leukemia or other neoplastic disease, which sometimes also causes widespread metaphyseal destruction.

In retrospect it is clear that *Pauline's* limp arm was the pseudoparalysis of Parrot, and was caused by severe pain due to metaphyseal destruction in the humerus. The hepatosplenomegaly is a consistent feature of congenital syphilis. Other findings seen in this condition that *Pauline* did not have include "snuffles," or rhinitis, skin eruption, and condylomas. She was, however, anemic, a common feature of patients with congenital syphilis.

Pauline's mother's rash during the third trimester probably represented the cutaneous manifestations of secondary syphilis. She was not diagnosed during the pregnancy, but after it became clear that her serologic test for syphilis was positive, she and the father were referred to the Public Health authorities for penicillin treatment and contact search. *Pauline* was treated with penicillin, also, and developed a febrile reaction and tachycardia characteristic of the Herxheimer reaction. This lasted for a short time and did not reoccur as treatment continued. The child has been followed in the outpatient department. As of the last visit, *Pauline* had begun to spontaneously move her left arm. The flagrant bone changes were reverting toward normal.

THE CLASSICS

Here are **the classics,** bone radiographs that time has served to sanctify and examiners to dignify by inclusion in all sorts of quiz presentations, examinations, and Boards. Topics that have been previously covered in *Exercises in Diagnostic Radiology, Volume 3, Bone* will not be covered in as much detail here.

FIGURE 181. Tina L.

Tina L., a 7 year old retired concert pianist, was unable to sign her unemployment compensation check because of stiff fingers. This radiograph was obtained (Fig. 181).

FIGURE 182. Phillip D.

Phillip D., a 1 year old food faddist, had a skeletal survey to confirm the clinical impression — which was . . . ? (This is an ancient case; currently we would shield the gonads.)

Mac W., age 1, another food faddist (Fig. 183).

FIGURE 183.   Mac W.

Tom S., age 9, might have been fed a very special diet that would have caused the bones to develop this radiographic appearance. However, he was fed a normal diet but developed these bone changes anyway (Figs. 184 and 185).

FIGURE 184.   Tom S.

FIG. 185

ANSWERS

Tina L.'s hand radiographs demonstrate soft tissue swelling surrounding the proximal interphalangeal joints. In addition the bones show generalized osteoporosis (reduced bone density). The margins of the carpal bones are irregular, indistinct, and reflect extensive bone destruction.

Tina has *juvenile rheumatoid arthritis.* Her symptoms began with stiffness in both hands. (A somewhat more classic presentation would have been fever, pain, and stiffness in the larger joints such as the knees or elbows.) The early radiographs showed only soft tissue swelling, but the current films show advanced changes of juvenile rheumatoid arthritis.

The radiographic changes are due to chronic inflammation, with thickening of the synovium that surrounds the joints, and destruction of the cartilage and eventually the bone. Hyperemia accompanies the inflammatory changes and is responsible for the deossification. Advanced bone age may occur in JRA; it is the hyperemia that is thought to cause this.

Tina has been treated with moderate success with aspirin and cortisone and physical therapy. The deformity and limitation of range of motion of the fingers and hands seems to be at least stable at the present time.

Philip D. has extremely osteoporotic bones. The appearance of the bones has been stated to resemble ground glass. The epiphyses have a cortical margin that is well defined and relatively radiodense. This is a distinctive feature of this condition. The metaphyses are flared. Fractures occurring through the zones of provisional calcification result in chipped off "corners."

Philip has *scurvy.* This is caused by vitamin C (ascorbic acid) deficiency and was manifest clinically by bleeding gums and tenderness in the legs. *Philip* had been fed exclusively on boiled cow's milk without vitamin supplementation. Cow's milk has considerably less vitamin C in it than breast milk, and boiling it reduces the vitamin C content even further. When treatment was begun with vitamin supplementation, calcification of the periosteal hematomas occurred.

Mac W.'s bone radiographs demonstrate the dense metaphyseal bands associated with lead ingestion. One caution, however: the normal patient may have dense femoral and tibial metaphyses, especially around age 2 years. The proximal fibular metaphysis never is this dense normally, however. Other reliable places to scan in evaluating a patient for lead ingestion include the distal ulna, the inferior border of the scapula, and the iliac crest, in other words, sites of rapid endochondral ossification.

The dense metaphyseal band does not represent locally deposited lead; it is secondary to the effect of lead, which alters the trabecular architecture of the newly formed bone. It has been stated that the lead interferes with the balance between deposition and resorption of bone. There is continued deposition of bone which appears radiologically as a dense metaphyseal band.

FIGURE 186. Mac W.

Mac W. had recently eaten lead-containing paint which appeared as radiopaque debris in the colon (Fig. 186). The colon was emptied of its poisonous contents, and courses of chelation progressively removed lead from the body.

The bone disease is almost incidental and causes the patient virtually no problems. It's the CNS that takes the blow and the bones that give the clue.

Tom S.'s radiographs show widening of the growth plate accompanied by cupping and fraying of the normally smooth borders of the metaphyses. Defective calcification of the osteoid is reflected radiologically by increased distance between the metaphysis and epiphysis.

Tom has vitamin D resistant rickets, an inherited unresponsiveness to normal quantities of vitamin D. His diet contained a normal amount of vitamin D. When *Tom* received a diet massively supplemented with vitamin D healing occurred.

THE CLASSICS, PART TWO

FIGURE 187. Christopher T.

Christopher T., age 8, had suffered a trivial injury while playing baseball. He had thought that he had a "charley horse," but because the pain didn't diminish and *Christopher* began to limp, his mother brought him to the pediatrician. Included here is one of the radiographs of the thigh area (Fig. 187).

FIGURE 188. Cheryl S.

Cheryl S., 14 years old, appeared quite ill. For approximately two weeks she had pain and soft tissue swelling in the region of the midportion of the right humerus. Recently the swelling and tenderness became more than she could bear, and she was seen by her pediatrician, who admitted her immediately to the hospital with the provisional diagnosis of osteomyelitis (Fig. 188).

Seth P., was 17 years old when these radiographs were obtained (Figs. 189 and 190). His diagnosis had been established three years earlier on the basis of a cervical lymph node biopsy. He had received treatment, but back pain and symptoms of nausea, vomiting and decreasing appetite had recently occurred. These radiographs were followed by an upper G.I. series (Fig. 192). What are the possible diagnoses? Has *Seth* had back surgery?

FIGURE 189. Seth P.

FIG. 190

ANSWERS

The radiograph of *Christopher's* femur (Fig. 187) shows an increased bone density of the distal half of the femur. Anteriorly, there is elevation and disruption of the periosteum accompanied by layers of periosteal reaction. Notice that there is tumor formation in the soft tissue. These are the findings of osteogenic sarcoma. Whether the increased density in the lower femur is due to new tumor formation or bone reaction to the process occurring is not known.

This malignant bone tumor has a very poor prognosis regardless of treatment. *Christopher* had an amputation of his leg; however, he developed lung metastases several months after surgery and died less than one year after the osteogenic sarcoma was discovered.

Cheryl S.'s clinical condition suggested osteomyelitis. She had the classic findings of inflammation: swelling, heat, redness, and loss of function. The radiograph of the humerus (Fig. 188) shows a mottled appearance to the mid-diaphyseal region indicating that a destructive process has permeated the bone. This area of involvement is accompanied by lamellae of periosteal reaction anteriorly and posteriorly. The lamellae of periosteum are sometimes referred to as having an "onion peel" appearance.

Because of the clinical impression of osteomyelitis, *Cheryl* was operated upon and the lesion was drained and biopsied. The pathology report was *Ewing's sarcoma.*

This is a malignant bone tumor thought to arise from the blood-forming elements. Its symptoms, signs, and radiographic appearance resemble osteomyelitis to a striking degree. The treatment of choice is radiotherapy. The prognosis is better than with osteogenic sarcoma. *Cheryl* has just completed her radiotherapy. There is not yet any evidence of metastases in the lungs or elsewhere, but it is still too soon to predict whether the radiotherapy was successful.

The differential diagnosis of periosteal reaction is important. Below (Fig. 191) is a child with periosteal reaction seen along the lateral aspect of the lower femurs. This child has leukemia. Here is a list of *some conditions that may cause periosteal reaction.*

Benign
1. Osteomyelitis
2. Bone infarct (think of sickle cell anemia)
3. Caffey's disease (infantile cortical hyperostosis)
4. Treated scurvy (due to ossification of subperiosteal bleeding)
5. Hypertrophic pulmonary osteoarthropathy (think of cystic fibrosis)
6. Osteoid osteoma
7. Gaucher's disease (not common)
8. Trauma

Malignant
1. Osteogenic sarcoma
2. Ewing's sarcoma
3. Eosinophilic granuloma (histiocytosis X)
4. Leukemia
5. Other primary and metastatic tumors of bone

FIG. 191

Seth's spine radiographs (Figs. 189 and 190) show that the eleventh and twelfth thoracic vertebrae as well as the first and second lumbar vertebrae are exceedingly radiodense. The third lumbar vertebra has patchy areas of increased radiodensity within it. The lucent area seen on the AP projection extending from the center of T 11 to L 2 is caused by surgery—a laminectomy. *Seth* has Hodgkin's disease which has involved the spine and caused spinal cord compression. A laminectomy was needed to decompress the spinal cord.

Blastic changes in the bone are uncommon in the pediatric population. They are seen however in Hodgkin's disease, medulloblastoma, osteogenic sarcoma, and occasionally leukemia. Lytic metastatic deposits, on the other hand, are seen very frequently, especially in neuroblastoma and leukemia.

Seth's upper G.I. series (Fig. 192) demonstrated separation of loops of small bowel accompanied by fixation and imprint formation or indentation on the serosal surface. This is due to involvement of the mesentery with Hodgkin's disease. The initial chest radiograph (Fig. 193) revealed massive mediastinal lymph node enlargement. The diagnosis of Hodgkin's disease was proved by cervical lymph node biopsy. *Seth* had radiotherapy and chemotherapy.

FIGURE 192.   Seth P.

FIG. 193

FIGURE 194. Shawanda T., June 21

FIGURE 195.   June 30

MORE PERIOSTEAL REACTION

Shawanda T., age 7, a black girl with sickle cell anemia was seen because of pain in the right arm of two days' duration.

Radiographs of her arm (Fig. 194) showed soft tissue swelling, expansion of the marrow space (thinned cortex), and fine periosteal reaction. These radiologic features are consistent with a bone infarct, and *Shawanda* was admitted to the hospital. A bone marrow aspiration documented salmonella osteomyelitis. On June 30, a second radiograph was obtained which showed permeative, moth-eaten changes in the humerus accompanied by a more extensive periosteal reaction. With antibiotic therapy, the child slowly improved.

Here is a common problem: the differentiation of bone infarct from osteomyelitis in sickle cell anemia. Radiologically these may appear exactly the same, and clinical and bacteriologic factors must form the basis for their differentiation. Children with sickle cell anemia are subject to both illnesses. The osteomyelitis is often caused by one of the salmonellae.

Other bone changes in sickle cell anemia include expansion of the medullary space due to an increased volume of red marrow. There is an exaggerated prominence to the bony trabeculae. Softening of the superior and inferior endplates of the vertebrae allows the nucleus pulposus of the discs to cause a characteristic indentation best seen on the lateral view of the spine. There is also an increased incidence of aseptic necrosis of the femoral head and other epiphyses. A curious entity is the "hand-foot" syndrome in which there are infarcts of the small bones of the hands and feet. Radiographs show periosteal reaction of the small tubular bones.

AND STILL MORE . . .

Jack C., age 3 months, had been irritable for about four days. He had also had a low-grade fever and soft-tissue swelling which surrounded the mandible and both forearms.

The AP view of the mandible shows a "new" layer of bone along the mandible. Normally the roots of the molars are within 2 or 3 millimeters of the exterior of the mandible in this age group. Here the new bone has almost doubled the thickness of the mandible (Fig. 196).

There is another x-ray finding seen on this radiograph: periosteal cloaking of the left clavicle. Similar findings are present in the radius and ulna on each side (Fig. 197).

These are the radiographic findings of **infantile cortical hyperostosis,** or **Caffey's disease.** This condition occurs in infants under age five months. The etiology is unknown, but infection, allergy, toxins, drugs, and hereditary factors have been suggested. The bones most commonly involved are the mandible, clavicle, ribs, and long bones of the extremities. Changes of **infantile cortical hyperostosis** are not seen in the phalanges or in the vertebral bodies.

The differential diagnosis radiographically includes the trauma X (battered child) syndrome and infection, such as syphilis. Usually the pattern of bone involvement (the mandible is most frequently involved) suggests the diagnosis.

Although most patients heal without specific therapy, steroids have been used. Some patients may develop a chronic form of this condition and demonstrate bony bridges between the ribs or radius and ulna.

The disease seems to be less common now than in the 1950's for unknown reasons.

FIGURE 196. Jack C.

FIG. 197

FIGURE 198.   Dick C.

FIGURE 199.   Dick C., Frogleg position

PROBLEM

Dick C., age 3, was noticed to be limping for about three days. Initially, his mother thought that he might have had pain in the right knee, but subsequently she thought the pain was centered in the right hip. The pediatrician found slight tenderness in the hip region and limitation of range of motion accompanied by

muscle spasm. He obtained these radiographs (Figs. 198 and 199).

The AP and "frog leg" lateral hip views show flattening of the right femoral epiphysis with irregular areas of rarefaction between areas of increased bone density. The right femoral neck is slightly broader than the left.

This is Legg-Perthes disease, which is ischemic necrosis of the capital femoral epiphysis. This condition is more common in boys. Its peak incidence is about age 7, but children as young as 2 years old have been seen with Legg-Perthes disease. Ischemic necrosis of the hip is also seen in association with Gaucher's disease, sickle cell anemia, hypothyroidism, steroid therapy, and in late stages of treatment of congenital hip dislocation.

The early radiologic manifestations of Legg-Perthes disease are an increase in the apparent joint space and fullness of periarticular soft tissue planes. A subchondral lucency then develops in the epiphysis. This lucency is crescent-shaped and in the next stage is followed by areas of dense bone separated by lucent areas composed of fibrous tissue. The femoral head appears to be dissolving into several fragments. It is flattened and the femoral neck is widened. When repair begins, gradual reconstruction of shape is seen with diminution in size of the lucent areas.

Notice the left hip in the "frog leg" projection. There is a lucent crescent in the joint space between the acetabulum and the epiphysis. This is gas that accumulated in the joint space as Dick's hip was gently manipulated into the frog leg position. Caused by diminished pressure in the joint during manipulation, it outlines the thickness of the articular cartilage. This is a "gas arthrogram" or the "vacuum phenomenon." The formation of a gas arthrogram in the hip has no specific significance by itself.

SKELETAL DYSPLASIAS

For many pediatric radiologists, the most difficult conditions to categorize are the skeletal dysplasias. This group of maladies comprises the inborn diseases that are reflected in unusual patterns of bone size and/or shape. The radiologist soon learns that it is necessary but not sufficient to memorize one pattern of bone malformation for one disease. The patterns change as the patient grows. In addition, in some of the dysplasias there is a spectrum of involvement from mild to severe. In general it is a sterile exercise (and frequently boring) to try to deduce from a set of radiographs alone the condition responsible for the changes. The history, physical examination, and genetic pattern in the family, studied together with the radiographs, make an exciting diagnostic problem, and in this context a few of the more common skeletal dysplasias will be presented here.

What do we mean by skeletal dysplasias? In general, they are inherited, although many occur by spontaneous mutation. Dr. Philip Rubin has suggested that the pattern of altered bone growth reflects the site of major derangement such as the epiphysis, growth plate, metaphysis or diaphysis.

In this section we are also going to discuss and illustrate some of the **mucopolysaccharidoses.** There are at least six conditions included in this general term: Hurler syndrome (MPS I), Hunter syndrome (MPS II), Sanfilippo syndrome (MPS III), Morquio syndrome (MPS IV), Scheie syndrome (MPS V), and Maroteaux-Lamy syndrome (MPS VI). These conditions have in common excessive storage in many tissues and urinary excretion of certain acid mucopolysaccharides.

There is another group of connective tissue disorders that show altered bone growth and/or mineralization, which, together with the clinical information, form a recognizable pattern. This group of diseases includes Marfan's syndrome, homocystinuria, and fibrodysplasia ossificans progressiva, etc.

Why put so much effort into cataloguing such rare and apparently hopeless conditions? The answer depends upon one's orientation. For the researcher studying cartilage growth, the patients with achondroplasia, hypochondroplasia, and achondrogenesis are models of abnormal cartilage cell growth. For the clinician caring for the patient with homocystinuria, it is quite important to know that arteriograms are to be avoided: patients with homocystinuria develop thromboses and may die. For the genetic counselor, it is important to differentiate diastrophic dwarfism which is inherited as a recessive trait, from achondroplasia, an autosomal dominant condition.

Lastly, for the patient, evidence is accumulating that metabolic abnormalities may be correctable in at least some of these conditions. For example, the altered metabolism of fibroblasts from patients with the Hurler syndrome is corrected by adding the missing enzyme to the culture fluid. The next problem is to find an effective way of administering the enzyme to the patient.

THE CLINICAL APPEARANCE OF FOUR DWARFS

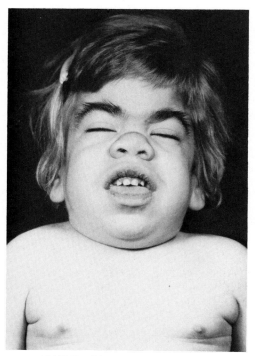

FIGURE 200.   Hurler syndrome

The following illustrations are dwarfs with skeletal dysplasias including the Hurler syndrome, or MPS I (Fig. 200); the Morquio syndrome, or MPS IV (Fig. 201); achondroplasia (Fig. 202); and pycnodysostosis (Fig. 203). (These are not the same patients whose skeletal surveys are seen on the following pages.)

The *Hurler syndrome* is inherited as an autosomal recessive trait. The patient illustrated here has the characteristic large head and prominent forehead. The nose is broad and the cheeks are puffy. If the eyes were open, corneal opacification could be seen. The tongue is enlarged and the lips are thick. The facial features are generally coarse. Examination of the abdomen would reveal hepatosplenomegaly. This child had stiff joints and a gibbus or hunchback deformity of the thoracic spine.

The *Morquio syndrome* is also inherited as an autosomal recessive trait. The patient pictured here is an adult. (The scale is in centimeters.) She demonstrates the striking dwarfism (patients with the Morquio syndrome are rarely more than four feet tall), and lumbar lordosis. Her thoracic cage has a large AP diameter.

The upper extremity is proportionally more shortened than the lower extremity. The knees are held in the genu valgum position (knock-knees). Unlike the Hurler syndrome, in which the joints are stiff, the Morquio patients have increased range of motion. This patient was quite normal mentally. Some patients become troubled with deafness as they grow older.

FIGURE 201.   Morquio syndrome

FIGURE 202. Achondroplasia

Achondroplasia is the most common type of dwarfism. It is inherited as an autosomal dominant trait, but seven out of eight cases occur as new mutations. Clinically these patients have a large head with frontal bossing. The nasal bridge is shallow. The chest and abdomen may be normal, but sometimes the abdomen appears protuberant. The gluteal region is prominent because of exaggerated lumbar lordosis; the upper and lower extremities are equally shortened and the fingers are stubby. The mental capability usually is normal, dull normal, or slightly more retarded.

Pycnodysostosis, an uncommon cause of dwarfism, is inherited as an autosomal recessive trait. This young lady still had open anterior and posterior fontanelles. This illustration shows the characteristic receding chin, about which more will be said later. The girl was just under five feet tall. She had short fingers with dished out, or spoon-shaped nails. Her problem clinically was that minimal trauma resulted in fractures. She was normal mentally.

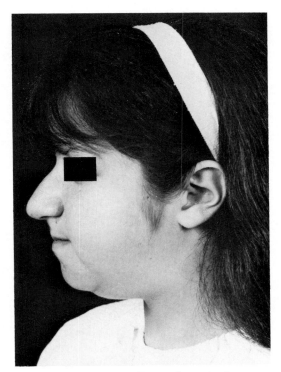

FIGURE 203. Pycnodysostosis

THE HURLER SYNDROME

FIG. 204

Of the six mucopolysacchari-doses, the Hurler syndrome occurs most frequently and is the most widely known. This child was 3 years old when these radiographs were made. At birth, the child seemed normal. The mental deterioration and grotesque facial features were present by the end of the first year.

The chest radiograph shows ribs that are wider than the interspaces. There is a characteristic narrowing near the vertebral column (paddle ribs). The heart may become enlarged when mucopolysaccharide deposition occurs in the myocardium and the valves. When the cardiac enlargement compresses the left lower lobe bronchus, atelectasis results as seen here. (There is also a plaque of atelectasis in the right upper lobe.) One of the frequent problems seen in the **Hurler syndrome** is recurrent pneumonia.

The hand radiograph demonstrates delayed ossification of the carpal bones, proximal pointing of the second through fifth metacarpals, and lateral enlargement of the metacarpals and phalanges. The distal ends of the radius and ulna are angulated obliquely so that they slant toward each other.

FIG. 205

The skull radiograph (Fig. 206) demonstrates the characteristic thickening of the skull base, large cranial vault, frontal bossing, fusion of the sutures, and a "J-shaped" or "omega" sella turcica. (The J-shaped sella is seen in a number of conditions including the normal infant. Actually it refers to depression of the sulcus chiasmaticus and planum sphenoidale, leading to a fancied resemblance to the letter J. It was shown by Dr. E. B. D. Neuhauser that arachnoid cysts are responsible for the formation of the J-shaped sella in the **Hurler syndrome.**) Notice that the mandible is short and the third molars are seated on the ramus.

The vertebral bodies (Fig. 207) have a concave posterior scalloping with pedicles that are longer than normal. The first lumbar vertebra is hypoplastic and situated posterior to the other vertebrae, thereby creating a gibbus deformity (hunchback). There is a tongue or beak of the inferior aspect of the upper lumbar vertebrae that protrudes anteriorly. This is a characteristic finding.

The radiograph of the pelvis (Fig. 208) reveals flared iliac wings and constriction of the body of the iliac bone with an almost imperceptible dimple (or "spicule") at the lateral margin of the acetabulum. This leads to subluxation of the hips. There is also bilateral coxa valga and delayed ossification of the capital femoral epiphyses.

FIG. 206

FIG. 207

FIG. 208

THE MORQUIO SYNDROME

FIG. 209

FIG. 210

FIG. 211

The patients with the Morquio syndrome differ from those with the Hurler syndrome in several important ways. The Morquio patients are usually normal mentally, whereas the Hurler patients are profoundly and increasingly retarded. The Morquio patients excrete keratin sulfate in the urine; the Hurler patients excrete dermatan sulfate and heparan sulfate. Both are strikingly dwarfed. The Hurler patients have marked corneal opacification, but this is milder in the Morquio patients. The Hurler patients do not survive nearly as long as the Morquio patients. In fact, one of the original patients described by Morquio was 54 years old in 1971! The patient seen here was 16 years old when these radiographs were made.

The chest (Figs. 209 and 210) has a marked pectus carinatum deformity and an increased AP diameter. The ribs are wide, especially anteriorly, and don't project over the sternum (on the lateral view).

The wrists are swollen and the hands are malformed (Fig. 211). Delayed ossification is seen. Other features of the hand radiograph include small carpal bones and proximal pointing of the second through fifth metacarpals. Because the ulna is shortened, there is ulnar deviation of the hands. Compare these radiographs with those of the other dystrophies.

FIG. 212

All of the vertebrae are flat-tened—platyspondyly. The lateral view of the cervical spine (Fig. 212) shows that the odontoid process is absent. The atlas is held close to the occiput, and upon flexion the atlas slips anteriorly over the axis. It is not surprising that one of the common causes of death is atlanto-axial dislocation, resulting in spinal cord compression.

In the lower dorsal and upper lumbar spine (Fig. 213) there is an anterior beak in the *middle* of the vertebral body. (In the Hurler syndrome the anterior beak is seen in the inferior or *hind* part of the vertebral body. M = middle = Morquio. H = hind = Hurler).

The pelvis (Fig. 214) shows marked narrowing of the iliac body. The acetabula are not well formed, and the hips are dislocated. The capital femoral epiphyses undergo changes that resemble aseptic necrosis and then eventually disappear. The femoral necks show a valgus deformity and become widened and fragmented.

FIG. 213

FIG. 214

ACHONDROPLASIA

FIG. 215

This patient was 7 months old at the time these radiographs were made. The view of the lumbar spine (Fig. 215) is almost diagnostic of achondroplasia because the distance between the pedicles decreases between the first and fifth lumbar vertebrae. Normally the interpediculate distance increases in this region. A lateral view of the lumbar spine would show shortened pedicles. It is not surprising that nerve root compression is seen frequently in patients with achondroplasia because of the diminished volume of the spinal canal.

The pelvis (Fig. 216) has squared iliac wings with a very narrow greater sciatic notch. The acetabular roofs are not quite horizontal.

FIG. 216

The long bones of the extremities (Fig. 217) are shortened, and their metaphyses flare. The epiphyses of the distal femurs appear to be sunken into the metaphyses. This change will develop in the proximal tibial epiphyses as well. In older children the fibula is longer than the tibia; this may result in inversion of the feet.

The base of the skull is foreshortened, while the membrane-formed vault is relatively large. The frontal region is characteristically prominent. The foramen magnum is small and is usually hidden in the normally positioned Towne's projection (Fig. 219). Some of the patients with achondroplasia develop mild hydrocephalus, probably of the communicating type. The hydrocephalus has been ascribed to the small foramen magnum, but the actual mechanism is probably much more complex.

The hands have a stubby shortened appearance. If the middle and ring fingers are separated, the term "trident hand" is used.

FIG. 217

FIG. 218

FIG. 219

FIG. 220

PYCNODYSOSTOSIS

FIG. 221

FIG. 222

The last of the skeletal dysplasias to be discussed here is pycnodysostosis. This condition is characterized by short stature (rarely are the patients more than five feet tall), dense bones that fracture easily, skull and mandible anomalies, and hypoplasia or absence of the terminal phalanges.

The base of the skull (see Figs. 221 and 222) appears thick. The sutures are widely separated, the fontanels are large, and sometimes wormian bones are seen. The sinuses are frequently poorly developed. The angle of the mandible is straight (Fig. 221).

The long bones (Fig. 223) are dense as seen in the distal radius and ulna. The hand radiograph also shows the striking hypoplasia of the distal phalanges and lack of the ungual tufts. The finger nails are frequently spoon-shaped and clubbed.

Clinically, fractures are the biggest problem. Trauma that wouldn't be remembered in a normal child causes fractures in children with pycnodysostosis. Unlike patients with osteopetrosis, anemia is not a problem.

This condition is interesting because it is now thought that the artist Henri de Toulouse-Lautrec suffered from pycnodysostosis. The evidence is reviewed in an article by Drs. Pierre Maroteaux and Maurice Lamy (J.A.M.A. 191:715–717, 1965). They point out that skeletal injuries prevented Toulouse-Lautrec from horseback riding, and his attentions were directed toward painting quite early. He suffered two known fractures from insignificant trauma. His fingers were very short and stubby and his height was 4'2".

One of the important features of pycnodysostosis is the appearance of the head. The mandible is small; Maroteaux and Lamy speculate that Toulouse-Lautrec grew a beard to cover his receding chin. The skull is large with open sutures and fontanelles. Most of the pictures of Toulouse-Lautrec show him wearing a hat (Fig. 224). It is thought that he wore a hat to protect the open fontanelles.

The parents of patients with pycnodysostosis frequently are related, since pycnodysostosis is inherited as an autosomal recessive trait. Toulouse-Lautrec's parents were first cousins. There are no known radiographs, and therefore no absolute proof, but on the basis of parental consanguinity, short stature, skull configuration, stubby fingers, and the history of fractures, it seems likely that Henri had pycnodysostosis.

The short fellow is Henri.

(This figure courtesy of Knud W. Jensen, Director of The Louisiana Art Gallery, Humlebaek, Denmark)

FIG. 223

FIG. 224

QUIZ

FINAL EXERCISE, REVIEW AND ACROSTIC

Find among the following 15 illustrations the one that best tallies with each of the items below on this page, then enter the *letter-designation of the figure* in the blank following the *corresponding historical item below*. When you have successfully completed the acrostic, you will have a comment we hope you'll make as you close the book.

ATTENTION: Figures may be used once, several times or not at all.

1. Child with a complication of sickle cell disease ...._____

2. Child who presented with a history of bloody diarrhea without pain for six weeks......................................._____

3. Baby with roentgen evidence for high small bowel obstruction ...._____

4. Baby with roentgen evidence of low small bowel obstruction ...._____

5. Child with colicky right flank pain and hematuria for 24 hours..._____

6. Child with episodes of diarrhea, fever, right lower quadrant pain, and tenderness ...._____

7. Child with cough and roentgen evidence for a posterior mediastinal mass......................................._____

8. Child with a right lower quadrant tender mass............._____

9. Child with plate-like atelectasis in the usual position of the minor fissure, secondary to the child's major problem_____

10. Child with cough and roentgen evidence for croup........_____

11. Child with unilateral ureteral obstruction and hydronephrosis ...._____

12. Child with projectile vomiting....................................._____

13. Child with midline abdominal mass but no symptoms..._____

14. Child with cough and roentgen evidence for left lower lobe collapse ...._____

15. Child whose chest film shows rib erosion....................._____

16. Child with six months' cough and evidence for an endobronchial foreign body.._____

17. Child whose intravenous urogram shows rotation of both kidneys ...._____

18. Newborn with choking and coughing upon first feeding_____

19. Child with cough and steatorrhea ...._____

FIG. L

FIG. P

FIG. A

FIG. C

FIG. D

FIG. G

FIG. S

FIG. Y

FIG. W

FIG. Y

FIG. H

FIG. I

FIG. T

FIG. H

Page 157

FIG. I

ANSWERS TO QUIZ

ANSWERS

1. Gall stones in sickle cell disease .... W

2. Ulcerative colitis .... H

3. Double bubble in duodenal obstruction .... Y

4. Unused colon, dilated small bowel .... T

5. Ureteral calculus at ureterovesical junction .... H

6. Regional enteritis I

7. Ganglioneuroma .... S

8. (Same as 6) I

9. (Same as 7) compression atelectasis .... S

10. Croup C

11. (Same as 5) .... H

12. Hypertrophic pyloric stenosis I

13. Fused (horse shoe) kidney L

14. Left lower lobe collapse .... D

15. (Same as 7) .... S

16. Nail in the bronchus intermedius .... P

17. (Same as 13) L

18. Esophageal atresia with atelectasis upper lobes .... A

19. Cystic fibrosis .... Y

(G was not used but shows a pleural effusion in a baby with staphylococcal pneumonia.)

INDEX

(NOTE: This is not really a formal index at all! Rather, it is simply meant to help you find something you want to see over again. Page numbers in **boldface** refer to page on which illustration may be found; those in lightface refer to discussion in the text.)

Abscess, retropharyngeal, **7,** 8
Achondroplasia, **139,** 139, **144,** 144, **145,** 145
Angiomatosis, encephalofacial, **94, 95, 96,** 96
Anus, imperforate, **64,** 64, **65,** 65
Aphthous stomatitis, **74,** 75
Appendicitis, **38, 40,** 40
Aqueductal stenosis, **112,** 113
Arthritis, rheumatoid, juvenile, **126,** 128
Artifacts, **103,** 103
Ascariasis, **69, 70,** 70
Aspiration of foreign bodies, **2,** 4, **7,** 8
Atelectasis, 4, 10
Atresia, choanal, **58,** 59
    duodenal, **66,** 67

Battered child syndrome (Trauma X syndrome), **117,**
    118, **120,** 120, **121,** 121
Bicuspid aortic valve, 21
Bladder, exstrophy of, **80, 82,** 82
Bowel obstruction, neonatal, **72, 73,** 73
Bronchial obstruction, **2, 4,** 4
Bronchiectasis, **2, 4,** 4

Caffey's disease, **135,** 135
Calculus formation, **80, 82,** 82
Choanal atresia, **58,** 59
Coarctation of the aorta, **20,** 21, **26,** 27
    adult (post-ductal), 21
    infantile (pre-ductal), 21
Colitis, ulcerative, **51, 53,** 53
Craniopharyngioma, **101,** 101
Craniosynostosis, **104, 106,** 106
Crohn's disease, **50,** 52
Croup, **5, 6,** 8
Cystic fibrosis, **30,** 31, **42,** 44, **45,** 45
Cystitis, 45
Cytomegalic inclusion disease (CID), **98, 100,** 100

Dextrocardia, mirror-image, **18,** 19
    situs solitus with, **18,** 19
Diaphragmatic hernia, **33,** 35
Down's syndrome, 19
Duodenal atresia, **66,** 67
Dysphagia, 6, 8
Dysplasia, fibrous, monostotic, **111,** 111

Ectopia, renal, crossed, **76,** 78
Emphysema, **30,** 31

Encephalocele, anterior, **114, 115,** 115
Encephalofacial angiomatosis (Sturge-Weber
    syndrome), **94, 95, 96,** 96
Enteritis, regional, **50,** 52
Eosinophilic granuloma, 110
Epiglottitis, acute, 8
Epilepsy, idiopathic, **102,** 103
Esophageal obstruction, **3,** 4
Esophagus, "lye burn" of, **74,** 75
Ewing's sarcoma, **130,** 132
Exstrophy, of bladder, **80, 82,** 82

Fracture, of distal left tibia, **123,** 123
    of radius and ulna, **122,** 122
    skull, **116,** 118

Ganglioneuroma, **9,** 10, **11**
Granuloma, eosinophilic, 110

Hand-Schüller-Christian disease, 110
Hemangioma, port-wine, **94,** 94
Hernia, diaphragmatic, **33,** 35
Hirschsprung's disease, **61, 63,** 63
Histiocytosis X, **108, 109,** 110
Hodgkin's disease, **131, 133,** 133
Horseshoe kidney, **76,** 78
Hurler syndrome, **138,** 138, **140,** 140, **141,** 141
Hyaline membrane disease, **32,** 34
Hydronephrosis, bilateral, **79,** 79, **81, 83,** 83
Hyperostosis, cortical, infantile, **135,** 135
Hypertrophic pyloric stenosis, **46,** 48

Idiopathic epilepsy, **102,** 103
Ileal stenosis, **60, 62,** 62
Imperforate anus, **64,** 64, **65,** 65
Infantile cortical hyperostosis (Caffey's disease), **135,** 135
Intracranial trauma, **117,** 118
Ischemic necrosis, of capital femoral epiphysis, **136,** 136

Kidney, horseshoe, **76,** 78
    pelvic, **77,** 78

Laryngotracheobronchitis, **5, 6,** 8
Lead poisoning, **127,** 128, **129,** 129

Legg-Perthes disease, **136,** 136
Letterer-Siwe disease, 110
"Lye burn" of esophagus, **74,** 75

Malrotation, complications of, **47,** 49
Meningocele, **84, 85,** 85
Meningomyelocele, **84, 85,** 85
Mongolism, 19
Monostotic fibrous dysplasia, **111,** 111
Morquio syndrome, **138,** 138, **142,** 142, **143,** 143
Mucopolysaccharidoses, 137

Necrosis, ischemic, of capital femoral epiphysis, **136,** 136
Neuroblastoma, **86,** 88
  metastatic, **89, 90,** 90, **91,** 91
Neurogenic tumors, **9,** 10, **11**

Obstruction, esophageal, **3,** 4
Osteogenic sarcoma, **130,** 132
Osteogenesis imperfecta, **97,** 97
Osteomyelitis, salmonella, **134,** 134

Pelvic kidney, **77,** 78
Pneumonia, 15
  lower lobe, **39,** 41
  staphylococcal, **28, 29,** 29
Polyps, juvenile, **69, 71,** 71
Premature synostosis, **104, 106,** 106
Pseudoparalysis of Parrot, **124,** 125
Pycnodysostosis, **139,** 139, **146,** 146, **147,** 147

Reflux, vesicoureteral, **81, 83,** 83
Retropharyngeal abscess, **7,** 8
Rheumatoid arthritis, juvenile, **126,** 128
Rickets, **127,** 129

Sagittal synostosis, of skull, **105,** 107
Salmonella osteomyelitis, **134,** 134
Sarcoma, Ewing's, **130,** 132
  osteogenic, **130,** 132
Scaphocephaly, **105,** 107
Scurvy, **126,** 128
Septal defect, ventricular, **25, 26,** 27
Sickle cell anemia, **39,** 41
Skull, fracture of, **116,** 118
  sagittal synostosis of, **105,** 107
Staphylococcal pneumonia, **28, 29,** 29
Stenosis, aqueductal, **112,** 113
  ileal, **60, 62,** 62
  pyloric, hypertrophic, **46,** 48
Sturge-Weber syndrome, **94, 95, 96,** 96
Synostosis, premature, **104, 106,** 106
  sagittal, **105,** 107
Syphilis, congenital, **124,** 125

Tetralogy of Fallot, **24,** 24
"Toddler's fracture," **123,** 123
Tonsillitis, **5,** 6
Toxoplasmosis, **99,** 100
Tracheo-esophageal fistula, distal, **54,** 56
  isolated, **55,** 57
Trichobezoar, **68, 70,** 70
Tuberculosis, primary, **12, 13,** 14
  pulmonary, **13,** 14
Tumors, neurogenic, **9,** 10, **11**

Ulcerative colitis, **51, 53,** 53
Upper respiratory infections, **12, 13,** 14

Ventricular septal defect, **25, 26,** 27
Vesicoureteral reflux, **81, 83,** 83

Wilms' tumor, **87,** 88